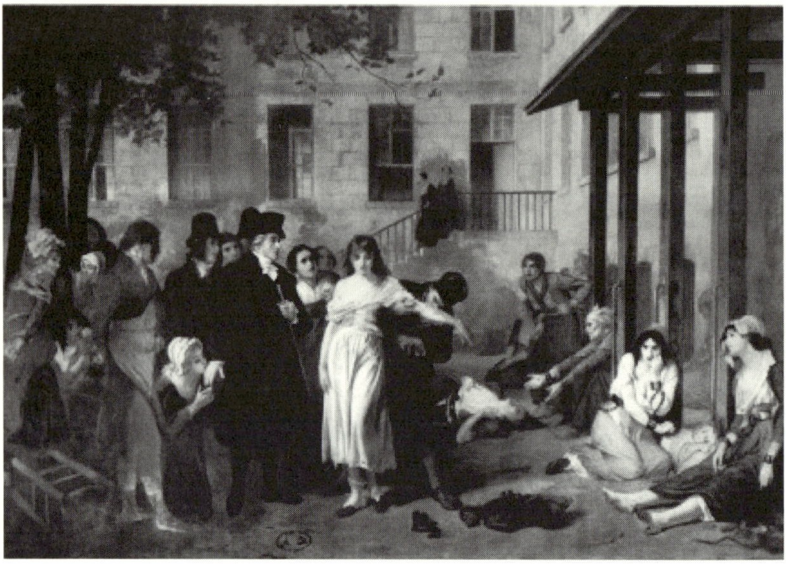

Dr, Philippe Pinel at the Salpêtrière, 1795, by Rober-Fleury. Pinel is removing the chains from patients at the Paris Asylum for Insane Women.

Dr. Edenharter's Dream

How Science Improved the Humane Care of the Mentally Ill in Indiana 1896–2012

Lucy Jane King, MD
Alan D. Schmetzer, MD

Portraits and drawings by Jan Royce

ISBN: 978-0-9831994-0-3

Image of Dr. Amariah Brigham is engraved by H.B. Hall from a daguerreotype, available at "Images from the History of Medicine," United States Library of Medicine, National Institutes of Health. Portraits on back cover are by Jan Royce.

Hawthorne Publishing
15601 Oak Road
Carmel, Indiana 46033
(317) 867-5183
www.hawthornepub.com

Dedication

Dedicated to all of those patients treated during the progression of Dr. Edenharter's dream. They, too, have hoped for a better future.

Contents

Prologue

What's Behind This Book?

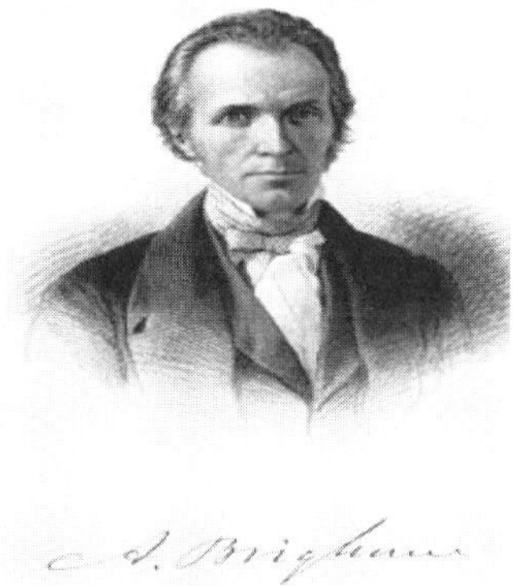

The treatment of the insane has ever varied with the philosophy and intelligence of the age. That they are better treated in modern times—more kindly and judiciously—is not owing to any increase of benevolence, but to an increase of knowledge.

Amariah Brigham, MD, July, 1847.

Dr. Brigham was one of the founding members of the The Association of Medical Superintendents of American Institutions for the Insane, which eventually became The American Psychiatric Association (APA). He was also the inaugural editor of the APA's official journal *The American Journal of Insanity* which we know today as *The American Journal of Psychiatry*. Like many of his colleagues in this country, Dr. Brigham was convinced of the treatability of psychiatric disorders. While this was not by any means an exclusively American belief, it is a potent philosophy which opens the door to all the future in this field.

Dr. Brigham's viewpoint quoted above embodies and implies this simple and direct thought: that the best hope of the treatment of mental disorders is the careful and methodical *scientific* unraveling of the secrets of psychiatric disorders and the measuring of the outcomes of various treatment approaches one against another.

This firm conviction forms both the philosophy behind and the content of this book.

1
The Ideas and Plans of the Superintendent

Central State Hospital I

In 2012 as this book was being finished, a world-class center for psychiatric and neurological disorders was in the final stages of completion on the Methodist Hospital campus of Indiana University School of Medicine, Indianapolis. A companion $45 million neuroscience research building was also being completed to provide together an exceptional national model for the treatment of the mentally ill through modern science.[1]

The new complex will be a center for studying and treating such disorders as schizophrenia, bipolar disorder, panic disorder, Alzheimer's dementia, alcohol and drug dependence, and autism spectrum disorders using the latest technology for the human genome. Planners envisioned scientists investigating the workings of brain structures using functional magnetic resonance imaging (fMRI) and other non-invasive studies of brain activity in living patients. Researchers on the ever-developing campus will be undertaking behavioral observations of human volunteers and laboratory animal models of disease, all with the goal of improving the treatment of—even finding cures for—Indiana residents suffering from psychiatric disorders.

Such were the plans as the reality of completion neared, with this book part of the celebration. The occasion allowed the authors to imagine the dedication of this precedent-setting complex. With much solemnity, officials will assuredly be giving speeches about the promise of today for mental health. The scientists will be sharing their hopes for the future. Some may mention the commendable history of psychiatric treatment in Indiana. Few of those paying tribute at the dedication of the complex, however, will be aware that these outstanding centers for brain research had their beginnings one hundred twenty years ago in a two-story brick building, state-of-the-art in brain science in its time, on the grounds of Central Indiana Hospital for the Insane, Indianapolis.

Called the Central Hospital Pathological Department, the sturdy brick research facility really was part of the reform of nineteenth-century medicine in America and a departure from a good deal of the care of the mentally ill at that time. Dr. George Edenharter, a pioneering physician in the care of the mentally ill, dreamed of, planned, and designed the Pathological Department building for studies of the brain at a time when public psychiatric hospitals were still pejoratively called "insane asylums," and the patients for whom they provided primarily custodial care were stigmatized by the public. Edenharter envisioned an auditorium for lectures and case presentations of patients from the hospital, a library of medical books and journals, laboratories for studies of blood and other body fluids and tissues, and facilities for autopsies. The building cost $12,000, a significant amount in those days.[2] The building of the Pathological Department established a direction of utilizing the best in science to improve the condition of the mentally ill in Indiana that has persisted through fluctuating fortunes until the present day.

Dr. Edenharter's vision was part of a revolution in medical care and education following millennia of ignorance. In the United States between 1885 and 1925, medical schools were modernizing to train physicians in newly developing knowledge in the medical sciences. In Indiana, with the opening of the Pathological Department, Edenharter created the equivalent of a department of psychiatry even before there was an Indiana University School of Medicine. The Central Indiana Hospital complex of buildings provided patient care, teaching, and research, the basic functions of any medical school department. New trends were clearly in the air.

Although there had been intermittent efforts at reform in the care of the mentally ill, at the end of the nineteenth century most psychiatric patients were still housed in large state institutions like Central Indiana Hospital for the Insane. Ideally care followed the "moral treatment" (better translated as improvement of morale) originated by Pinel in France in the late eighteenth century. It emphasized kindly relationships with patients, discussion of their social and psychological problems, purposeful activity, and pleasant surroundings. Much more likely was the reality of custodial care—or even worse, abuse—by untrained attendants. Coming to the facility as its new superintendent in 1893, Edenharter hoped to follow moral treatment methods and to train attendants in knowledge of the mentally ill and their treatment, but beyond that to discover specific treatments for specific diseases, treatments that might even lead to cure, a forward-thinking attitude for the time.

The Progressive era in American politics was reaching its peak, and the political atmosphere interfaced with the emerging medical revolution. In the 1890s state and local governments were beginning to regulate medical practice, and legislatures, funding agencies, and newly wealthy potential donors were taking careful looks at financial undergirding and sound and accountable management of hospitals before they bestowed their gifts.

Entrance to medical school increasingly required a college education; medical schools became divisions of universities, and the best medical school curricula now included two years of preclinical laboratory training in basic biological sciences and two years of clinical work on hospital wards and in clinics under the supervision of university faculty physicians. The goal of medical education became the use of up-to-date science to develop critical thinking in young physicians as they entered the practice of medicine.[3] Reforms were developing more slowly, however, in the specialty of psychiatry. Edenharter was determined to change that. He believed the scientific method was the key to helping patients in his new assignment at Central.

His deep commitment to the mentally ill was heartfelt. Although dealing with an institution with a growing population of several hundred patients, a small staff, and the usual limitations of budgets, Edenharter insisted on compassionate treatment of those entrusted to the state institution he was to head. He exhibited "warm and loving sympathy with the inconceivable sadness of mental affliction. . . .whenever questions of efficiency, economy, or expedience arose, always the one striking, all-absorbing impulse of his heart was to put foremost the consideration and defense of the helpless ones within his care."[4] In a notice posted for staff in 1897, Superintendent Edenharter wrote:

> As the insane are confined to our care for protection as well as treatment, no person will be employed here in any capacity who is not prepared to do all in his or her power to aid us in this. Any ABUSE or NEGLECT of a patient coming under their notice, it will be their especial duty to report it AT ONCE to the Superintendent who can ALWAYS be seen for this purpose. Should it at any time appear that ABUSE or NEGLECT has been witnessed and not brought to the notice of the Superintendent, or medical officer, it will result in the IMMEDIATE dismissal of all the parties concerned, the so-called "honor" that prevents reporting the abuse of a helpless insane person not being wanted for employment at this Hospital.[5]

He had cause for concern. There were 1,500 patients when Edenharter came to Central Indiana Hospital. Mistreatment of patients was always a problem in large public hospitals, and Central Indiana Hospital was no exception—even though physicians made "rounds" to visit their patients and to discuss cases with the ward nurses who had continuing contact with patients, and superintendents' wives, including Marion Edenharter, often acted as "matrons," assuming the role of an ombudsman who visited the patients on the wards and performed services such as replacing eyeglasses or providing a needed article of clothing.

Edenharter's eye quickly went beyond good and humane custodial care. Eager to research the structure of the brain and its relevance to psychiatric treatment, Edenharter made plans to build what he would call a Pathological Department building to house laboratory and teaching facilities on the far north end of the grounds of the hospital. It was to be the first building in the United States that included all three of the following characteristics: dedication to clinical and laboratory research in neuroscience, neuropathology, and psychiatry; association with a hospital so that research and clinical findings could be correlated; and provision of teaching for medical schools and physicians throughout the region.[6] These included older "proprietary" schools run by a few physicians who charged fees for lectures as well as the developing medical departments at Indiana University, Purdue University, and other colleges in the state. All medical students and physicians in the state would be invited to attend case conferences and lectures by guest professors from institutions such as the Chicago medical schools and the Johns Hopkins University, one of the preeminent universities in building a modern medical school.

In 1894, as the new and innovative Pathological Department was being planned, attention in Indianapolis began to focus modestly on the man at the state hospital who was seeking new methods for the treatment of the "helpless insane" with the tools of science. Edenharter had been born in Piqua, Ohio, to parents who had emigrated from Germany in the mid-nineteenth century as part of the influx of German immigrants to the lower Midwest at a time of political turmoil in Europe. When he was a young man, the family moved to Indianapolis. His father was a cabinet maker and, for a time, George worked as a cigar maker to earn money for medical training. He also served on the Indianapolis city council for four years. Traveling a path characteristic of medical education in the nineteenth century, he apprenticed to a physician in Indianapolis in the 1880s, then attended one of the better local proprietary medical schools, and, finally, practiced general medicine. After his medical training was completed and he had established a practice, he married his childhood sweetheart, Marion Swadener. They would have one son.

In 1890 Edenharter was selected as medical director of the City Hospital in Indianapolis, where he built a reputation as a gifted administrator. In 1893 the board of trustees of Central Indiana Hospital for the Insane asked him to be its superintendent.[7] Dr. and Mrs. Edenharter and their son, like most public hospital superintendents and their families, came to live on the grounds of the hospital. Edenharter's own compassionate instincts and American training and experience were enhanced by continuing study of new trends in European medical research and practice. He was literate in German and able to study scientific publications from Germany, then the leader in medical science in Europe. He was in touch with leading psychiatrists in the United States like Drs. Ira Van Gieson and Adolph Meyer.[8] In line with the changes in medical education and research in America at the time, he saw a brighter future for education, research, and patient care in psychiatry than had been available to him as a young physician and, as he worked with architects and the Board of Control of the hospital to see it through construction on the north side of the grounds, envisioned the Pathological Department as a road to the future.

The Pathological Department building was dedicated December 18, 1896, under the auspices of the Marion County Medical Society.[9] President Carson of the Board of Control noted that construction had been "according to the ideas and plans of our superintendent Dr. Edenharter" and that it was completed "without leaving indebtedness standing against the State," most important, then as now, in legislative politics. In his address, Dr. H. M. Lash, president of the Marion County Medical Society, reflecting some of the controversies and cross-currents of the time, commented,

> Similar institutions have been wanting and have been reaching out for this very thing . . . In insane hospitals, especially in those of the East, considerable scientific research has been carried out, very much as you propose to carry it on here; but it has been done either under great difficulties or with deficient or self-furnished equipment by the physicians in charge . . . It has been hard, very hard indeed . . . to convince legislative bodies that insane people need anything beyond a place where they can be kept under proper and safe environment, have some food to eat, and a few clothes

> to wear. And even, in these matters they have been disposed, in too many instances, to be [ungenerous]. . . [10]

Also on behalf of the Marion County Medical Society, Dr. Henry Jameson, a supporter of building the Pathological Department, presented Edenharter with "the latest pattern of Bausch & Lomb's biological microscope, a perfected instrument, costing $150." Edenharter replied, addressing particularly the Board of Control,

> I feel that I have simply done what any man in my position would have. I have worked to bring this institution to that point where it might safely be said that we were at least attempting to inaugurate a scientific era in the treatment of these diseases: and when I say that I have given my time and made many personal sacrifices in order to accomplish this end, I do not state the case too strongly. . . I feel tonight as if I had been the means of placing something in the hands of the profession whereby they may benefit humanity. I feel as if I may have added one brick, at least, to the structure of the medical profession . . .
>
> I hope that the work that will be done in this building will be upon the same broad plane that has been pursued in the construction of it; and we need have no fears hereafter of going to the East to be snubbed. The [mid] West has brains, and they are in the possession of the medical profession. I know from now on they will be used, and let them look to Indiana. Gentlemen, I heartily thank you, and I know that those of you who know me personally know that you need never fear to come out here at any hour of the day or night, and that you will receive a cordial welcome.[11]

Both politics and midwestern pride were evident at this early date. We now realize, as they did not, that the major impediment to fulfilling the lofty predictions of the dedication speeches of the brain study center was the fact that the technology of the day was inadequate to study the basic functioning of the brain. That would certainly impede the bright dream. Although the light microscopes like the one presented to Edenharter remain important even today in studying glass slides displaying very thin slices of stained tissue, they cannot view in detail the tiny spaces between brain cells (synapses) that later became recognized as crucial to understanding psychiatric disorders. At most, these microscopes magnify to about 2,000 times. Many later modifications of microscopy equipment allowed better visualization of the complexities of cells. For example, electron microscopes—large and expensive equipment—use electron beams rather than light rays to measure much tinier parts of carefully prepared cells, with magnifications up to 2,000,000 times. Synapses are visualized in detail. Later advances in methods and equipment for measuring brain chemistry—e.g. chromatography to separate chemicals and spectroscopy to study chemicals by means of absorbed or emitted light—helped to identify the chemical messengers in the brain, neurotransmitters, that traverse synapses to carry messages from one cell to the next. Computers to analyze data from high-tech equipment have revolutionized research. Although he could not have known in his day, it was synapses and neurotransmitters that Edenharter was looking for but had no equipment or methodology to find.

Even so, there was promise for useful studies at Central Indiana Hospital. What could be studied at autopsy by dissection of organs and study of tissue under the light microscope at the time were many of the so-called "organic" brain diseases or those "due to a general medical condition." Brain tumors, head injuries, abuse of alcohol or drugs, accidental poisoning, and congenital malformations of the brain might cause memory loss, decreased intellectual function, even hallucinations and delusions, as well as other symptoms such as disorientation to time and decreased perception and awareness of the environment. In addition, there were no antibiotics at the time, and infections of brain tissues were common and often caused psychiatric symptoms similar to those caused by other medical conditions. Many of the individuals suffering from organic diseases and brain damage caused by infection were admitted to psychiatric hospitals. On these Edenharter and the other physicians concentrated. By comparing clinical symptoms in a live patient in the wards with his or her later autopsy findings, and accumulating data on many such cases, some idea could be gained of which parts of the brain were associated with what symptoms and which disorders caused what kinds of damage to the brain. This would be most important in the later research of Max Bahr and Walter Bruetsch.

How would the specific day-by-day scientific work be done at this new medical landmark facility in Indiana? At the dedication Dr. Ludvig Hektoen, professor of pathology at Rush Medical College in Chicago, who would later become well known as head of the Department of Pathology at the University of Chicago, editor of several medical journals, and a widely published researcher, spoke of promising new technology.[12] Dr. Hektoen's address was titled "An Historical Outline of the Methods of Anatomical and Pathological Investigation of the Nervous System." He described the methods that had been devised in the nineteenth century by many investigators in many countries to preserve tissue sections of body organs, stain them to highlight specific cells and nerve fibers, and study them using light microscopes. Recent discoveries were making it possible to study the cells and nerve tracts of the brain itself. The Pathological Department was equipped to use all these methods. Dr. Hektoen concluded,

> It is the especial object of laboratories of this kind, if inaugurated right, to enlarge knowledge by a careful study of their rich material along the recognized lines of neuroanatomical and pathological investigation, and to utilize the methods and opportunity now available for researches bearing upon the relation of the insanities to structural changes in the nerve cells. In this and all its work may this laboratory succeed.[13]

The Pathological Department's equipment for autopsy dissections of the brain and microscopic study of tissue sections would allow the facility to remain state-of-the-art for a half century.

All of these promising ideas would depend on funding to carry out the research. That was the practical part of the dream, and Edenharter believed he was the man to handle that aspect of the work also. Before becoming a hospital administrator, Edenharter had been involved in local politics. Although he maintained a strictly nonpartisan perspective after being appointed to head City Hospital and Central, he kept up contacts with the legislature, urging the importance of the work at the Pathological Department in educating physicians.[14] Early on he had to face political challenges head on. There was a great deal of controversy about the building of the Pathological Department in the mid-1890s, centering around the concern that such an elaborate and expensive laboratory was unnecessary for a state hospital for the insane. Local medical lore passed down through the years has it that Edenharter was able to disguise needed equipment for the new building in the existing budget. Ultimately, he managed to construct it with very creative use of existing funds and little financial support from his friends in the state legislature. As the department continued its work, Edenharter developed the academic administrator's necessary skills and grew adroit in writing the equivalent of grant requests in his day—getting money from the legislature. He did get help from his friends there, but for the actual building of the new facility, he was largely on his own.

Officials organized tours of the new building, and the press and public began to see its innovative scientific space and equipment for themselves. Edenharter had worked carefully with the architect in the design of the building, using the skills he had developed at the city hospital—and probably early in life from his craftsman father—to design a truly modern facility for the efficient use of the latest laboratory techniques. Once the building was opened in 1896, pictures of the building and floor plans of its layout were included in subsequent *Annual Reports to the Governor.*

The Indianapolis News reported on December 16, 1896, that

the building was the first of its kind in Indiana hospitals, "and the first anywhere of like equipment, for the apparatus has been largely devised by Superintendent Edenharter. It meets all the requirements of pathologists, and besides the special advantage it will be to the physicians of the hospital it will furnish the students of the medical colleges of Indiana an opportunity to study diseases of the brain and nerves under the most favorable conditions."

A Trip Back in Time: 1896

A visitor entering the Pathological Department in its opening phase would see that all the woodwork in the building was oak. On the right on the first floor was a modest parlor with a fireplace. Also on the first floor was a room where families who had permitted autopsies on patients who had died in the hospital of as yet untreatable medical disorders (e.g. infectious diseases) could bring their own clergy to have a funeral for their loved ones at no cost to them. Behind closed doors beyond the parlor was a bacteriology laboratory with glassware to prepare cultures of bacteria from specimens from patients with illnesses and a small oven to incubate preparations of bacteria. Sterilizing ovens as well as scales to weigh chemicals for preparations to be used in the laboratories were housed along one wall of an adjoining room.

Beyond the entrance hall in a room with a skylight was a round built-in oak table with space open in its center where an instructor could stand and perform dissections for students to examine organs, examples of which were in jars of preservative in the glass-fronted cabinets around the walls.

The auditorium on the first floor had cane-bottomed chairs arrayed in semicircular tiers rising to the back of the room. The autopsy room was off to the left. In an age before electronic, or even electrical, dictating equipment, a metal tube ran from the autopsy room through the ceiling to the second floor. A small room there had a desk and a large ledger. The physician performing the autopsy "dictated" his findings through the tube, and the doctor on the second floor copied them in the ledger with a pen dipped in an inkwell. Records were kept in this second floor room.

Edenharter and his medical staff could integrate findings from clinical examinations and observations in the hospital, results of laboratory tests performed in the laboratories, and autopsy results to form a better picture of patients' illnesses. Records of many patients could be correlated to achieve better understanding of a given illness and its outcome. To the right of the auditorium, the visitor would find offices for the doctors.

Upstairs were two laboratories: one with equipment for chemical studies of blood and urine specimens and microscopic examination of blood cells and another for preparation and study of tissue, preserved and sliced into very thin sections that could be stained and mounted on microscope slides to reveal individual cells. Microscopes were aligned along a laboratory bench in front of windows that added more light to the gooseneck lamps that provided illumination for microscopes. Down the hall was a room with a special camera apparatus that could take enlarged pictures of microscope slides as well as prepare 3 by 4 inch glass slides for projection on a screen during lectures. There were shelves for books and journals in a conference room.

Small amenities were provided. There was a lavatory on each floor. In one corner of the auditorium was a faucet and paper cups that provided iced drinking water from blocks of ice placed in a cabinet above it for faculty giving lectures.

To realize the goals of the Pathological Department to disseminate information about new ways to treat psychiatric disorders long-term, it would be desirable, even necessary, to involve the teaching institutions in the state. Once the building was up and functioning, Edenharter focused on the teaching aspect of his goals. Central Indiana Hospital for the Insane was located in the largest city in the state, the capital Indianapolis, and was not far from Indiana University in Bloomington and Purdue University in West Lafayette. These universities were beginning to develop modern medical departments and to contest which would be chosen as the state medical school. Three proprietary medical schools in the state would eventually, in 1905, combine as the School of Medicine of Purdue University.

Meanwhile, Indiana University, which had a two-year medical school, began negotiating for clinical facilities in Indianapolis for the final two years of training. In 1906 the State College of Physicians and Surgeons in Indianapolis joined with Indiana University to conduct the last two years in Indianapolis hospitals after two years of training in scientific subjects in Bloomington. In 1908 Purdue agreed to withdraw from medical education, and the Indiana University School of Medicine was opened in Indianapolis.[15] Edenharter brought groups of students from all of the medical schools in the state to the Pathological Department both before and after the consolidations.

Thus the Pathological Department initiated its work and involved staff to do the actual research as they could, with teaching institutions to feed into the process and expand the work.

Fulfilling the promise of the planning and dedicatory years was not easy.

True, there was recognition during the period 1896–1910 that the work out at Central Indiana Hospital for the Insane was important. Later reports by the trustees and superintendent continued to supply reasons for the importance of the department. For example, the 1905 *Annual Report* issued by Superintendent Edenharter states,

> The wisdom of the establishment of this department is becoming recognized more and more as the work therein continues, and while at the time of its erection and establishment it was an entirely new departure in hospital management, yet today it is taken advantage of by the medical

> profession of the state and medical students receive therein a course of practical instruction with apparatus and facilities more complete than can be found in many medical colleges.

The superintendent also noted the importance of autopsies in educating medical students and physicians. The duty of the state included provision of this kind of education for physicians—it was not just important, it was their *duty*! Providing instruction to the physicians prepared them to recognize and help the mentally afflicted in their communities and increased their ability to deliver an intelligent judgment in insanity inquests, thus saving the state money by decreasing the number of persons annually committed to state institutions. Training would encourage medical students' interest in psychiatry and provide future staff for the hospital. The public would be educated about these matters as well by publications and lectures of the staff. But there were serious roadblocks to progress in significantly helping or curing the mentally ill through science, and these obstacles went beyond the fact that the technology they needed was not as yet invented. One difficulty was simply the lack of personnel time: the physicians were too busy to devote hours to research and teaching.

The wards at Central were full of people needing physicians' diagnosis and care. Edenharter had early on realized he would need help. He could not supervise or head up the research alone. In 1898 Edenharter had hired Dr. Max Bahr, an Indianapolis native and graduate of a local medical school. Bahr had served as chief resident physician at the Government Emergency Hospital in Washington, DC, where he saw patients from the Government Hospital for the Insane (St. Elizabeth's Hospital) and became interested in psychiatry. After assuming the position at Central Indiana Hospital, Bahr developed a detailed plan for careful clinical examination to be performed on all patients and began what were, in essence, epidemiological studies. He catalogued summaries of patients by gender and other demographic characteristics and by diagnosis, reporting first on over 300 patients and later on more than 2,600 patients. His findings were correlated with pathological findings in research reports published by the hospital, presented to the local medical society, and distributed to colleges and universities throughout Indiana. Such data provided a picture of sociological factors in disease, thus opening possibilities for understanding causes.

In 1908 Edenharter gave Bahr leave of absence for a year to study in Germany. Like Edenharter, Bahr was the son of German immigrants and fluent in German. Bahr's father was a musician who had played piano concerts to entertain the Kaiser's troops in the Franco-Prussian War and later became prominent in musical circles in Indianapolis, for example furnishing background music as James Whitcomb Riley gave poetry readings. When Bahr returned to Indianapolis in 1909 with a doctorate of psychological medicine from the University of Berlin, he became the first physician at Central Indiana Hospital with formal training as a psychiatrist. In Europe Bahr had studied the theories of the time, including those regarding prevention of, and medication and psychological treatment for, psychiatric illness.

But problems persisted in recognition of the importance of science-based improvements in treatment in Indianapolis. As the first decade of the twentieth century ended at Central, statistics showed the patient population was growing significantly, while physician-to-patient ratio had not. There was also the inevitable dissention in the ranks of the physician/researchers themselves. In 1912 one of those physicians, Dr. Edward Kempf, told the Legislative Visiting Committee that few autopsies were being performed in the Pathological Department building. Some of them, he added, were inaccurate. Professional rivalry may have played into his critical analysis and comments. Kempf, who later became a psychoanalyst in New York, was interested in long-term, intensive psychotherapy, not possible with the patient load of a physician at Central Indiana Hospital.[16] Edenharter had been displeased with Kempf's neglecting his total workload to spend time with a few patients testing out some of his theories and had rebuked his subordinate.

Kempf told the 1912 Visiting Committee that modern

treatments were not being used on the wards. He did exclude a couple of the physicians from his criticisms, including Bahr.[17] But the superintendent himself was implicitly the target of most of the testimony. Although Central Indiana Hospital for the Insane remained an integral part of the training of medical students and residents at Indiana University School of Medicine for several decades, Edenharter's dream of extensive psychiatric research was not fully realized during his tenure. Ever-increasing demands of patient care on the few staff physicians ultimately caring for more than two thousand patients kept staff busy on the wards as in any other public hospital. Obtaining funding was always a problem in view of legislative caution in spending tax money for psychiatric illnesses, which the public abhorred and stigmatized anyway. In addition, families were not always eager to give permission for autopsies of loved ones, so continuously available material for study was not easily obtainable. Professional jealousies and criticisms played into the mix to diminish the effectiveness of the facility's performance. The press could be either an ally or an enemy. All of these challenges to excellent psychiatric care would persist into the future.

When Edenharter died in 1923, Bahr became superintendent of what soon (1927) would be called simply Central State Hospital. He would take the promise of Edenharter's dream to a new level.

Notes

1. Indiana University-Purdue University Indianapolis News Center, published April 15, 2011.
2. C. Bonsett, "The Old Pathology Building," *Indiana Medical History Magazine* 1 (1975): 7–11.
3. K. L. Ludmerer, *Learning to Heal* (New York: Basic Books, 1985), 4–5.
4. Board of Trustees of Central Indiana Hospital, quoted in George Edenharter obituary, *American Journal of Psychiatry*, 81 (1924)155-7.
5. Reproduced in *Indiana Medical History Quarterly*,7(1981)13.
6. In the late nineteenth century, autopsies were not uncommon in state

psychiatric hospitals. Because no effective treatments were available for psychiatric disorders, patients often remained hospitalized for years. Few treatments were available for common infectious illnesses, cardiac problems, or other medical conditions. Patients in psychiatric hospitals not infrequently died with medical diseases. Autopsies and laboratory studies were carried out, usually in local general hospitals that provided such services for the psychiatric hospitals. Seldom were studies done comparing results from many patients to better understand disease. An exception was the Kankakee State Hospital in nearby Illinois, where there was a clinical pathology laboratory established by Dr. Adolph Meyer, the founder of modern American psychiatry. (E. Shorter, *A History of Psychiatry: From the Era of the Asylum to the Age of Prozac* [New York: John Wiley & Sons, 1997], 91–93.)
Departments of psychology in some universities and colleges had laboratories for the study of physiological psychology—measures of blood pressure, pulse, and the like under various psychological conditions. In January 1895 the well-known professor of psychology at Clark University, G. Stanley Hall, described the laboratory at McLean Hospital, associated with Harvard University Medical School. It consisted of five small rooms, devoted to physiological psychology studies, chemistry of body fluids, studies of blood cells, and autopsies. The entire hospital was to be relocated in the near future. (G. S. Hall, "Laboratory of the McLean Hospital Somerville, Mass.," *American Journal of Insanity* 55 [January 1895]: 357–64.) It became an outstanding facility in the twentieth century.

7. R. F. Stone, *Biography of Eminent American Physicians and Surgeons* (Indianapolis: Carlon and Hollenbeck, 1894), 155–56; J. P. Dunn, *Indiana and Indianans* (Chicago: The American Historical Society, 1919), 251–53.

8. About the same time that Edenharter was working in Indiana, Dr. Ira Van Gieson became director of the New York State Laboratory (later Institute), a central pathology laboratory to service all the state mental hospitals. He envisioned a multidisciplinary research facility. There were political and other controversies, and his vision was not realized until Dr. Adolph Meyer became director in 1902, moved the research institute to the grounds of a hospital, and added education to the functions of the hospital. The institute later became affiliated with the Columbia University College of Physicians and Surgeons. (L. C. Kolb and L. Roizin, *The First Psychiatric Institute: How Research and Education Changed Practice* [Washington, DC: American Psychiatric Press, 1993], 3–5; and S. Kety "Introduction," Kolb and Roizen, *The First Psychiatric Institute*.)

9. "Dedication of the Pathological Department of the Central Indiana Hospital for the Insane, Under the Auspices of the Marion County Medical Society, Friday Evening, December 18, 1896," *Indiana Medical Journal* 15 (January 1897): 277–85.

10. Ibid.

11. Ibid.
12. Biography of Ludvig Hektoen, "Ludvig Hektoen Papers: An Inventory of His Papers at the University of Illinois at Chicago Library of the Health Sciences," http://www.uic.edu/depts/lib/specialcoll/services/lhsc/ead/LHS-EAD-1b.html.
13. L. Hektoen, "An Historical Outline of the Methods of Anatomical and Pathological Investigation of the Nervous System," *Indiana Medical Journal* 25 (January 1897): 264–69.
14. *Forty-sixth Annual Report of the Trustees and Superintendent of the Central Indiana Hospital for the Insane, to the Governor* (Indianapolis: Wm. B. Burford, 1895) and *Forty-seventh Annual Report of the Trustees and Superintendent of the Central Indiana Hospital for the Insane, to the Governor* (Indianapolis: Wm. B. Burford, 1896).
15. C. J. Phillips, *Indiana in Transition: The Emergence of an Industrial Commonwealth, 1880–1920* (Indianapolis: Indiana Historical Bureau and Indiana Historical Society, 1968), 418–19.
16. M. Engel, "Psychoanalysis and Psychosis: The Contribution of Edward J. Kempf," *Journal of the American Academy of Psychoanalyis and Dynamic Psychiatry* 18 (1990): 167–84.
17. Indiana Commission on Public Records, "Central State's Medical Staff and the Emergence of Scientific Medicine, 1890-1920," http://www.in.gov/icpr/2719.htm.

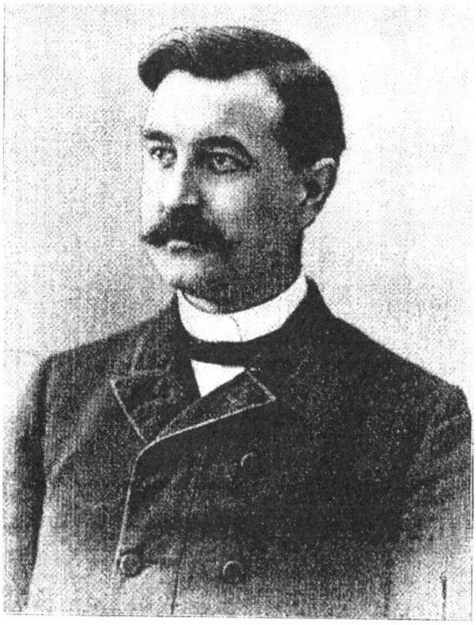

Dr. Edenharter was well known and respected in Indianapolis. Before becoming a hospital administrator, he served two terms on the city council and, in a race for mayor, lost by only a few votes in a city where the majority of voters were of the opposite political party.

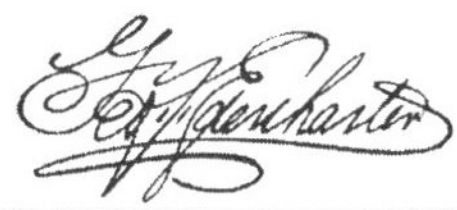

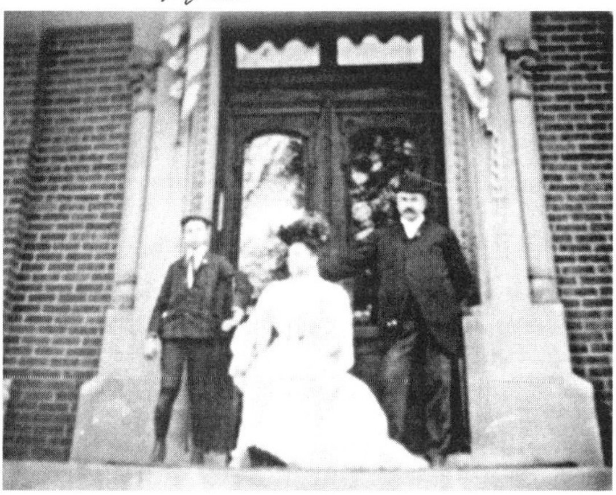

The Edenharters' son, Ralph(l), became a lawyer. As an adult he lived in Philadelphia.

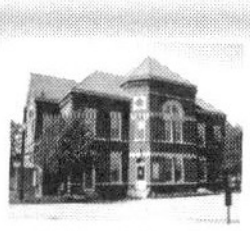

The former Pathological Department building is now the Indiana Medical History Museum. All photos of the Pathological Department and its personnel are courtesy of this institution.

Unless otherwise identified,portraits of historical and recent-day leaders in Indiana psychiatry and biological drawings are by Indiana artist Jan Royce. Photographs are from the authors' private collections or those of colleagues.

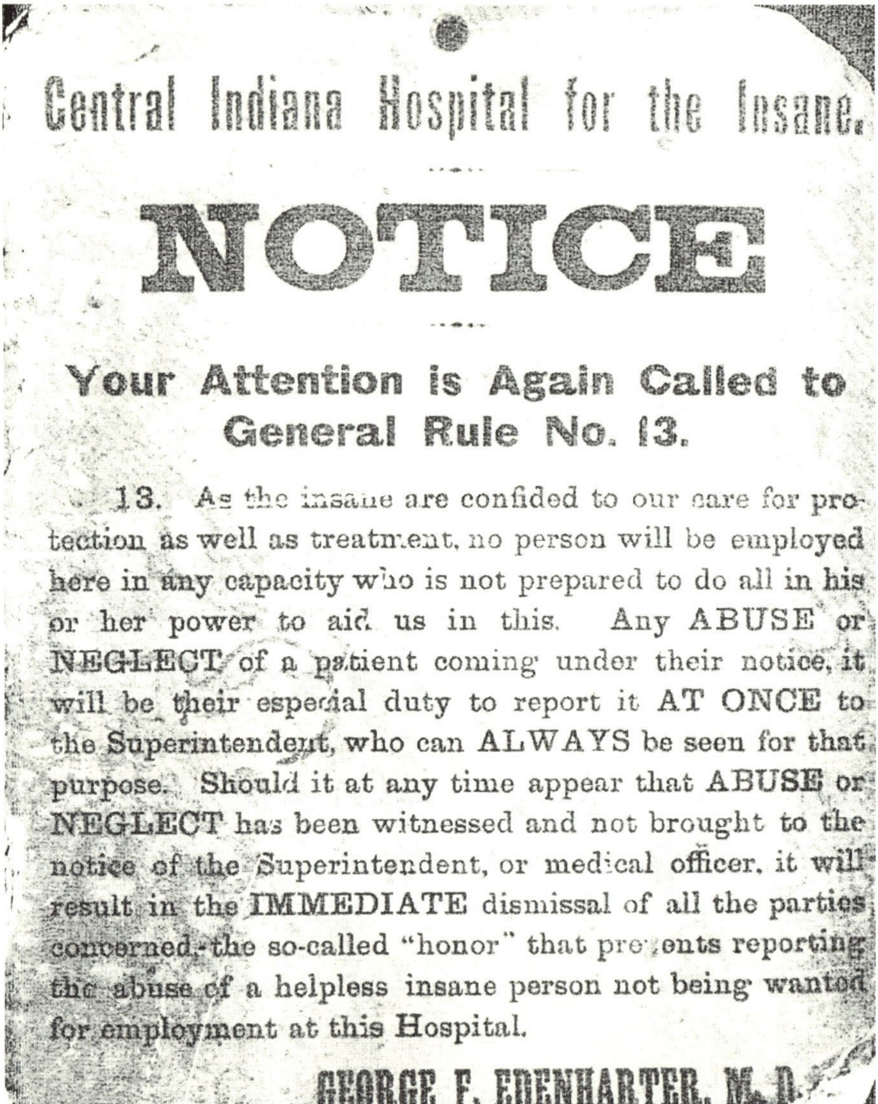

Central Indiana Hospital for the Insane.

NOTICE

Your Attention is Again Called to General Rule No. 13.

13. As the insane are confided to our care for protection as well as treatment, no person will be employed here in any capacity who is not prepared to do all in his or her power to aid us in this. Any ABUSE or NEGLECT of a patient coming under their notice, it will be their especial duty to report it AT ONCE to the Superintendent, who can ALWAYS be seen for that purpose. Should it at any time appear that ABUSE or NEGLECT has been witnessed and not brought to the notice of the Superintendent, or medical officer, it will result in the IMMEDIATE dismissal of all the parties concerned—the so-called "honor" that prevents reporting the abuse of a helpless insane person not being wanted for employment at this Hospital.

GEORGE F. EDENHARTER, M. D.

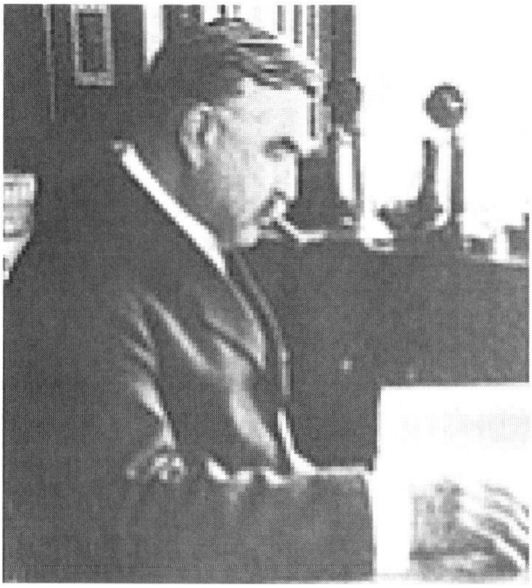

Superintendent George Edenharter in his office in mid-career.

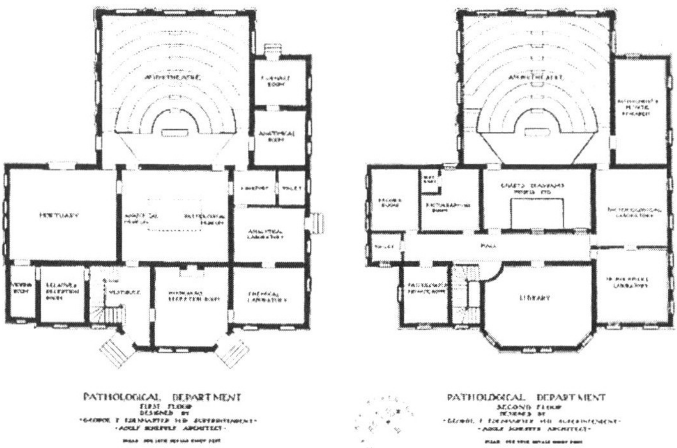

Pathological Department floor plan.

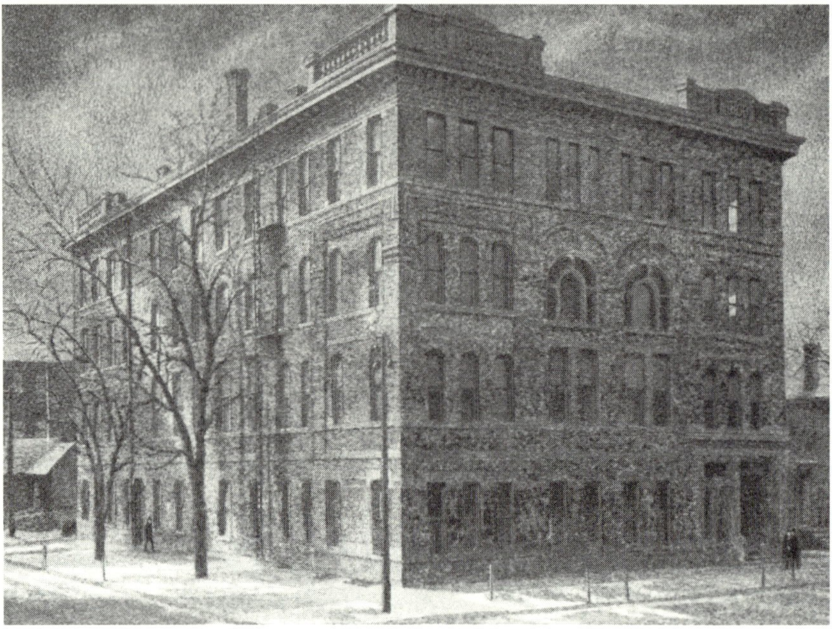

Courtesy Indiana Medical History Museum.

The history of Indiana Medical College in Indianapolis, shown here in a painting by Indiana artist Harry Davis, is typical of medical schools in the last half of the nineteenth century as reforms in medical education were beginning. It was founded in 1860 and located at the corner of what is today Senate and Market. In 1878 it merged with the College of Physicians and Surgeons to form the Medical College of Indiana. In 1905 it joined the medical colleges of Butler University, University of Indianapolis, and Fort Wayne College of Medicine to become the School of Medicine of Purdue University. It remained in Indianapolis throughout its life as a college and finally became a part of Indiana University School of Medicine in 1908.

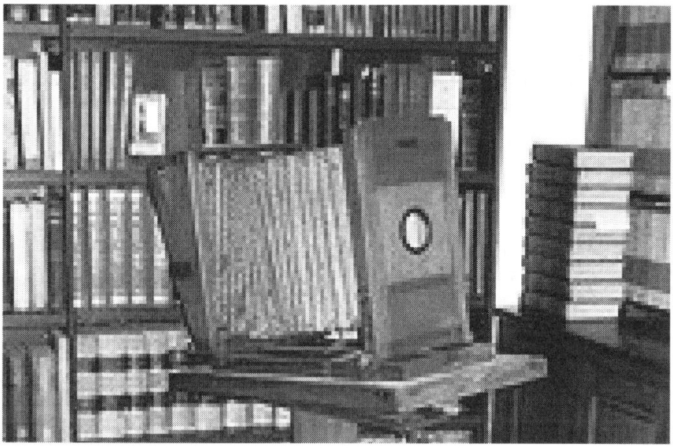

The photography laboratory at the Pathological Department allowed magnified microscope slides to be photographed and placed on 3¼x 4-inch glass plate slides to be shown in lectures. Students today download illustrations from the internet.

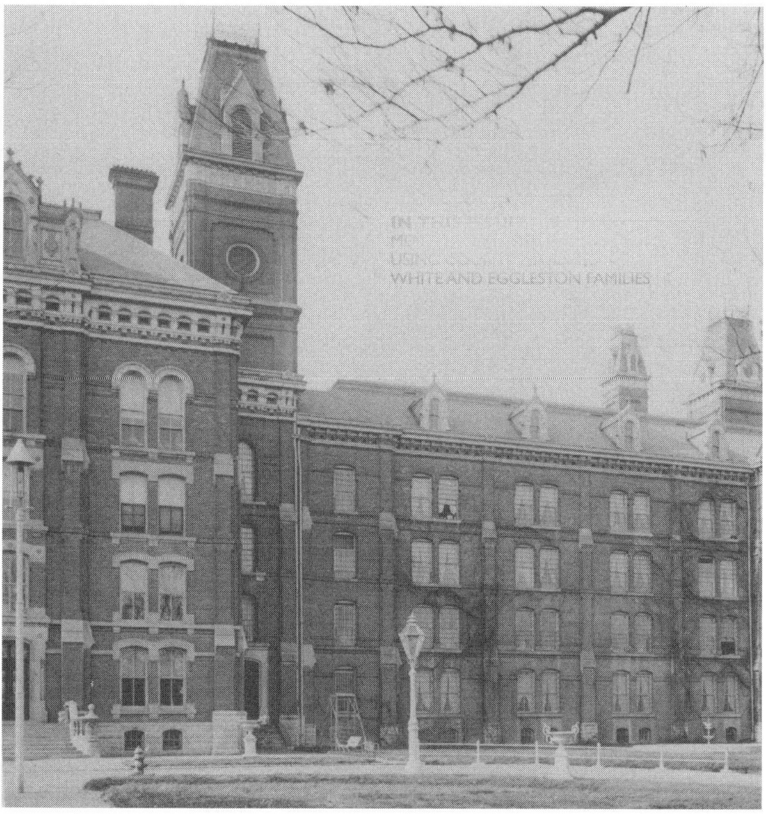

The Women's Building at Central Indiana Hospital for the Insane, called "Seven Steeples." It actually had eight steeples (three of which are seen here) but from any vantage point on the ground, only seven steeples could be seen.

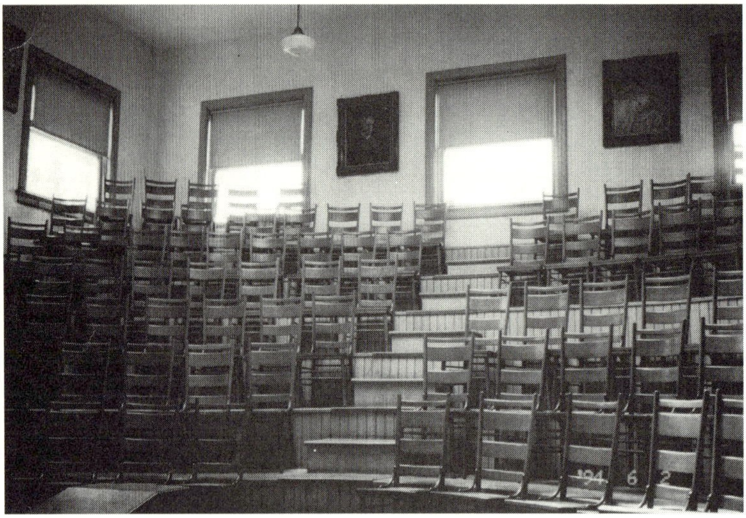

Auditorium seating in the Indiana Medical History Museum, about as it was.

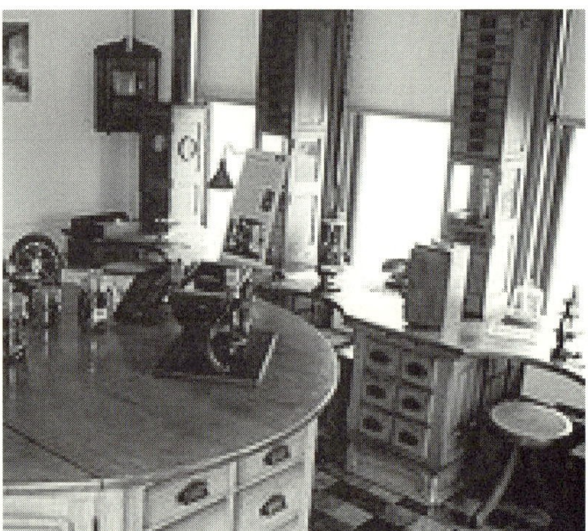

Histology (study of structure of cells, tissues, organs) laboratory where very thin tissue slices were stained and prepared for microscope slides. The arrangement of lighting and cabinetry shows Edenharter's skill in planning and design. The Pathology Department is restored in today's Medical History Museum.

2
The Best Possible Means of Benefiting the Incurable

Central State Hospital II

There had been continuing difficulty in keeping a pathologist long term at the hospital. Fortunately, in the early 1920s, Max Bahr met Dr. Walter Bruetsch, who was visiting relatives in Indianapolis. Bruetsch was born in Germany and was in the German army in World War I; injured and captured by the French, he was treated by the world-famous French neurologist, Joseph Babinski. Bruetsch had subsequently become a neuropathologist, trained in Germany and Switzerland. This meeting at a social gathering began a professional partnership of Bahr the clinician and Bruetsch the neuroscientist.

Problems that George Edenharter had faced in the 1890s continued to vex state hospital administrators in the new century. In spite of lectures in the community by Bahr and other professionals, the public continued to misunderstand and stigmatize patients with psychiatric disorders. These attitudes influenced voters' views as to how the state legislature allocated tax monies to state hospitals. Hiring trained staff or offering training for existing staff was difficult with limited funding, contributing to poor patient care in many hospitals that still housed several thousand patients each.

Edward Kempf's criticisms of Edenharter presaged a philosophical debate in American psychiatry in the first half to two-thirds of the twentieth century. Followers of Sigmund Freud and his associates and successors emphasized the importance of long-term psychotherapy. Those who were interested in research about the brain, as Edenharter had been, emphasized the biological aspects of psychiatric disorders. Until midcentury neither had discovered causes and cures of mental illness, but that didn't prevent heated arguments and the tendency to an either/or mentality—either psychological or biological factors, not both, were important, as the argument went. Nonetheless, state psychiatric hospitals had to do the best they could for the thousands of patients who came to their doors; they did not have staff time for long-term psychotherapy, and the many medications available today for psychiatric disorders had not yet been discovered. Specific treatments for mental illness were simply not possible.

There was one exception, however. Bruetsch and Bahr were among early investigators in the United States to study the first *effective* treatment for a *specific* psychiatric disorder. It was possible because the knowledge gained from the study of an infectious disease could be applied to the treatment of a psychiatric disease. It had been known since ancient times that some cases of severe mental illness would remit if the patient developed a high fever from an unrelated illness. In the last decade of the nineteenth century and the first decade of the twentieth century, it was determined that the specific illness that improved with high fever was "general paralysis of the insane" or "paresis," a late stage of syphilis, occurring years after the initial infection. *Treponema pallidum*, the organism causing syphilis, had been discovered in brains of patients with paresis, and blood tests for the illness had been developed early in the twentieth century.

In Germany Julius Wagner-Jauregg, who had discovered which psychiatric illness responded to fever, found the best method of artificially inducing fever to be use of a mild strain of malaria. Unlike other infectious diseases in this era before antibiotics, malaria could be cured—with quinine. After a period of malaria-induced fevers in patients with paresis, the malaria itself was cured. Of Wagner-Jauregg's first nine patients, six showed a "plainly favorable" outcome, and three of these were actively working at their normal occupations four years later. He received the Nobel Prize for this work in 1927.[1]

There were many patients with this disorder in psychiatric hospitals around the world, including Central State Hospital in Indianapolis. An untreated case of paresis ". . . was marked by increasing dementia, physical enfeeblement, and degradation of habits. The delusions, the grandiose fabrications, and the depressive ideas gradually died away leaving the patient in a state of apathy and inertia in which his mutterings would dimly recall fragments of his former delusions. His awareness of his whereabouts grew more and more dim . . . in the terminal stage, a shrunken and dilapidated shadow of his former self, he led a purely vegetative life. . .Very soon he had difficulty in getting about or even standing without support."[2] Death came to all but a small percentage of patients.

In their building on the grounds of Central State Hospital, Bahr and Bruetsch were among the first to implement and study the new treatment, and they soon reported on their first hundred cases. These included patients in all stages of paresis. When the paper was written, 25 had been discharged improved, of whom 21 had returned to their same or a similar occupation. An additional 12 were expected to be discharged soon. In other words, 37 (25 discharged and 12 to be discharged) of the 100 had returned to a level approaching normal function. In another 50 cases, little or no improvement was noted, 32 of them showing gradual decline. However, Bahr and Breutsch noted, "[p]reviously untidy patients attend to their personal cleanliness and keep themselves neat. Apathetic patients do a little work on the ward and have become helpful to the other patients. The attacks of excitement with very few exceptions have disappeared or at least have become less severe and the patients are as a rule easier to care for."

Five patients died during malaria therapy. Two deaths were attributed to malaria, two to complications of late-stage paresis, and one to pneumonia. Of the original 100 cases, 18 died within two weeks to eighteen months. Those who died within two weeks had late-stage paresis. Bahr and Bruetsch reviewed cases and reported autopsy results. In addition Bruetsch began a thorough study of autopsied cases to try to determine why the malaria treatment worked, a controversial question at the time about which many hypotheses had been proposed. Bruetsch developed his own theories about immune cells in the brain that attacked malarial parasites.[3]

However, theories about malaria became moot when penicillin became available to the civilian population after World War II. After a quarter century of the study of severe mental illness, Bruetsch was able to say about paresis, ". . . penicillin, if given in sufficient amounts, is superior to malaria therapy. I would not be surprised if this study means the end of the malaria treatment, which has never been an ideal way of treating general paralysis, but which was the *best possible means of benefiting this otherwise incurable brain disease*" [emphasis added].[4] It would still be a few years before antipsychotic medications would become available for serious psychiatric illnesses.

In the 1930s, when the malaria treatment protocol was at its height at Central under Bruetsch, psychiatry in America was slowly extending its search for treatment of the mentally ill into several new directions, some productive, some not. Training for psychiatrists greatly improved and formalized during the 1930s. The American Board of Psychiatry and Neurology, established in 1934, required a year of general medical internship plus three years of psychiatry (or neurology) residency after medical school and successful completion of day-long oral examinations in order to be a "board-certified" psychiatrist (or neurologist) and to present oneself as such to the public.

By this time the majority of psychiatrists were no longer serving as asylum superintendents. The specialty had been brought back into the mainstream of medicine. Psychiatrists had outpatient practices and treated patients with the newer psychoanalytic techniques or with behavior therapy or with some combination of theories and methods, using the medications available. For patients too ill to be cared for in the psychiatrist's office, there were private psychiatric hospitals or psychiatric units in general hospitals. Nonetheless, by the end of the decade, state institutions were taking care of over 90 percent of the hospitalized mentally ill—well over 400,000 individuals.[5] Central State Hospital was one of these institutions, and its patient care load day to day was heavy.

In the 1930s hypnotics ("sleeping pills") were used at Central State Hospital to improve sleep, sedatives to calm agitation, and stimulants to improve mood, although they did not greatly improve major depression. In the twenty-first century names and uses of medications prescribed for psychiatric disorders are commonplace. Whole textbooks for mental health professionals discuss antidepressants, antipsychotics, mood stabilizers, and anti-anxiety drugs. None of these were available in the 1930s or even the 1940s.

The division in American psychiatry at the time between "psychological" and "biological" concepts of causation and treatment involved two trends: the incorporation of perspectives from sociology and anthropology into psychotherapy and the use of "psychosurgery" and induced convulsions as biological treatments. Both the psychological and biological aspects were in this decade included in training and examinations of psychiatrists.

Psychiatrists trained in classical psychoanalytic theories were expanding those theories, too. Harry Stack Sullivan focused on interpersonal processes and the influence of the environment on individual development. Karen Horney brought a feminine perspective to theory and therapy. Erich Fromm saw man as an individual with many choices of action in any given social setting rather than a victim of predetermined instincts ("psychic determinism"). Ego psychology described the executive part of the personality (ego) as adapting to external reality as well as dealing with internal conflicts. Erik Erikson defined the stages of development and formulated a theory of individual development within a social matrix. At the same time behavioral therapists were expanding the classical conditioning of Ivan Pavlov (dogs salivate when a particular sound occurs) to clinical situations and ways of interpreting human behavior. In psychotherapy they tended to focus on current problems rather than childhood conflict, in fewer sessions than traditional psychoanalysts.[6] Bahr and Breutsch were aware of these crosscurrents and new directions, but most remained on the fringe of their studies and work with patients.

The biological scientists came into their own in specific ways. Advances in neurosurgery, such as the ability to cure some epileptic patients by removal of a damaged part of the brain, led to hope that "psychosurgery" might benefit patients with psychiatric disorders. After studying symptoms like emotional blandness of patients who had sustained injury to the frontal lobe (the "executive" part of brain just behind the forehead), António Egas Moniz in Portugal in 1935 postulated that cutting nerve tracts to this area would benefit patients with major depression and performed the first such surgery ("prefrontal lobotomy"). In the United States, Walter Freeman developed a method of cutting the tracts by inserting an instrument through the eye sockets. Although this treatment was utilized at the Logansport Hospital, records do not show it being utilized at the Pathological Department. It was largely discontinued as a treatment by the mid-1950s.

Manfred Sakel, treating opiate addicts in Berlin in 1933, observed that diabetic addicts were less anxious during opiate withdrawal when given insulin. After that some psychiatrists in the United States and elsewhere treated schizophrenia with insulin coma until antipsychotics became available in the 1950s. The antipsychotics were much more beneficial. An erroneous belief that patients with epilepsy never had schizophrenia led Ladislas von Meduna in Hungary to try convulsions induced by pentylenetetrazol (Metrazol) as a treatment for schizophrenia. Convulsions proved more helpful in the treatment of mood disorders than for schizophrenia, especially major depression. Insulin coma lowered brain sugar (glucose), and Metrazol convulsions decreased brain oxygen. Deficits in either of these crucial nutrients of the brain could prove dangerous. Like psychosurgery, these treatments became obsolete in the 1950s. A different focus dominated the studies at Central State Hospital.

The one treatment of all these "heroic" efforts that has continued to benefit a great many patients and was used at Central is electroconvulsive treatment (ECT, or electroshock treatment, EST). Paul Huston, chairman of the department of psychiatry at the University of Iowa medical school, reviewed hospital records and demonstrated that after the introduction of ECT, the average length of stay at the state hospital was reduced by months. Both depression and mania were greatly improved in many cases.[7]

ECT was a regular mode of treatment at Central during the 1940s. Bahr and Bruetsch studied national trends of treatment for schizophrenics with electrically induced convulsions and treated patients with this method. They then reacted to the subsequent finding that these treatments were more beneficial for patients with mood disorders. As with the malaria treatment of paresis, Bahr and Bruetsch always carried out follow-up studies to see which treatments were beneficial and which were not.

In many ways Bruetsch was decades ahead of his time. Technology in the 1990s made possible immunological methods that could study the questions he had asked about fever treatment of paresis and its effects on the brain.[8] His studies of the effects of streptococcal infection in the brain dealt with an area still being explored.[9]

In 1938 Central State Hospital was described in a report by the National Committee for Mental Hygiene about the twenty public hospitals located in ten states and the District of Columbia that were leading in psychiatric research. The report demonstrates that Edenharter's original grouping of research, hospital connection for clinical work, and teaching were still in operation:

> The Central State Hospital is the only one of the Indiana state hospitals active in research work. It has one of the largest and best-equipped neuropathological laboratories in the country for research in mental diseases. It is closely affiliated with the University Hospitals of Indiana University, and serves as a teaching center in psychiatry for Indiana University School of Medicine. The superintendent is professor of psychiatry and head of the department of nervous and mental diseases of the Medical School, and the director of laboratories is clinical professor of psychiatry. There is a

> training program for residents in psychiatry. . . The physical arrangements for laboratory work are excellent and well suited for research, a large two-story building [the Pathological Department] being used for this purpose. Pathological work is extensive . . . Three technicians are employed in addition to the pathologist. There is a library of 1,200 volumes. The laboratories were reorganized in 1931 after a visit by the director to all the important mental hospital laboratories in this country and abroad.
>
> ... Extensive investigations have been carried on in the histopathology of the psychoses with subacute bacterial and chronic rheumatic endocarditis and on the histopathology of neurosyphilis. In collaboration with the U.S. Public Health Service, Washington, D.C. and with the Coöperative Clinical Group a comparative study is being done of the various types of non-specific therapy. The director of the laboratories at this time (Bruetsch) is particularly interested in the frequency of chronic rheumatic brain disease found in [schizophrenia] patients. Another study deals with hypoplasia (underdevelopment) of the vascular system. . ."[10]

Bahr lectured to physicians and the public in Indianapolis about a variety of topics in psychiatry. He maintained close contact with state legislators to keep them informed about all that was happening at Central State—and the need for funds and support. He opened outpatient clinics for patients discharged from the hospital and added social services and occupational therapy for hospital patients. He lectured to law students to keep them informed about issues relevant to psychiatry that might impact their clients and court cases. Bahr was known for visiting with patients' families during visiting hours on Sunday afternoons.

The Pathological Department continued its excellent record, combining research, clinical connection, and teaching until after the Second World War. Bahr retired as superintendent of Central State Hospital in 1952 and died within the year. Within three years, medical students from Indiana University no longer came to Edenharter's Pathological Department building for lectures and laboratory demonstrations. But even now, in the twenty-first century, some of the original clinical reports and tissue specimens collected and preserved at the Pathological Department of patients who had Alzheimer's disease are being studied by researchers in the Department of Pathology at Indiana University School of Medicine for comparison with data from current patients in order to understand the development of the disease in the population over time.

By the mid-1960s, Bruetsch was the only one of the early physicians still working in the Pathological Department. Dr. Charles Bonsett, a neurologist, maintained an EEG laboratory and the Indiana Neuromuscular Research Laboratory there. In 1969, fearing that the Pathological Department was scheduled by state authorities for razing, several local physicians and other citizens including Bonsett, Dr. John U. Keating, Dr. Dwight W. Schuster, Dr. William M. Sholty, and Mrs. Donald J. White established a private, non-profit foundation to preserve the building. In 1971 the Pathological Department was rededicated as the Indiana Medical History Museum, a monument to Indiana's medical heritage. It was added to the National Register of Historic Places and to the Historic American Buildings Survey. In 1986 the state legislature granted the organization a ninety-nine-year lease for the building and the surrounding five acres.[11]

Central Indiana Hospital for the Insane and the Pathological Department building, under Edenharter's guidance, were the first neuroscience center in Indiana and a national model visited by psychiatrists from around the country. The Pathological Department's usefulness was over. It was time for two new facilities in Indianapolis to carry on the study of the science of mental illness and translate that into the best available treatment.

In 1952 the state of Indiana opened Larue D. Carter Memorial Hospital as a locale for treatment of acute psychiatric illnesses, clinical research about the newly discovered specific treatments for particular psychiatric disorders, and teaching of medical students and psychiatry residents. Sixty years after Edenharter's

Pathological Department was built, construction was started on the Institute of Psychiatric Research at Indiana University School of Medicine. When the building was dedicated in 1956, six researchers were already busy in their laboratories. These two buildings across the street from each other on the Indiana University School of Medicine campus became the second center for patient care, teaching, and research in psychiatry and neuroscience. They will be fully discussed in following chapters.

Notes

1. J. Wagner-Jauregg, "The Treatment of General Paresis by Inoculation of Malaria," *Journal of Nervous and Mental Disease* 55 (1922): 369–75; L. J. King, "The Best Possible Means of Benefiting the Incurable: Walter Bruetsch and the Malaria Treatment of Paresis," *Annals of Clinical Psychiatry* 12 (2000): 197–203.
2. E. Slater and M. Roth, *Mayer-Gross, Slater and Roth's Clinical Psychiatry*, 3rd ed. (London: Balliere, Tindall, and Cassell, 1969), 523.
3. M. A. Bahr and W. L. Bruetsch, "Two Years' Experience with the Malarial Treatment of General Paralysis in a State Institution," *American Journal of Psychiatry* 84 (1928): 715–27.
4. W. L. Bruetsch, "Penicillin or Malaria Therapy in the Treatment of General Paralysis? (A Clinico-anatomical Study)," Diseases of the Nervous System 120 (1949): 368–71.
5. L. J. King, "A Brief History of Psychiatry: Millennia Past and Present—Part II, Institutional Treatment," *Annals of Clinical Psychiatry* 11 (1999): 57–54.
6. L. J. King, "A Brief History of Psychiatry: Millennia Past and Present—Part III, Psychosocial Theories and Therapies," *Annals of Clinical Psychiatry* 11 (1999): 99–107.
7. L. J. King, "A Brief History of Psychiatry: Millennia Past and Present—Part IV, Neurobiological Theories and Treatments," *Annals of Clinical Psychiatry* 11 (1999): 175–84.
8. R. W. Keane and W. F. Hickey, *The Immunology of the Nervous System* (New York: Oxford University Press, 1997).
9. S. E. Swedo, "Pediatric Autoimmune Neuropsychiatric Disorders Associated with Streptococcal Infections (PANDAS)," *Molecular Psychiatry* 7S (2002): 24–25. There is continuing investigation of the effects on the brain of early life infections using studies of the body's immune responses unavailable to Bruetsch: A. S. Brown and E. J. Derkits, "Prenatal Infection and Schizophrenia: A Review of Epidemiologic and Translational Studies," *American Journal of Psychiatry* 167 (2010): 261–79.

10. National Committee for Mental Hygiene, *Research in Mental Hospitals* (Albany, NY: Boyd Printing Company, 1938), 38.
11. L. Bachelder, "'Inaugurating a Scientific Era': The Pathological Department, Central Indiana Hospital for the Insane (1896–1996)," pamphlet, Indiana Medical History Museum archives.

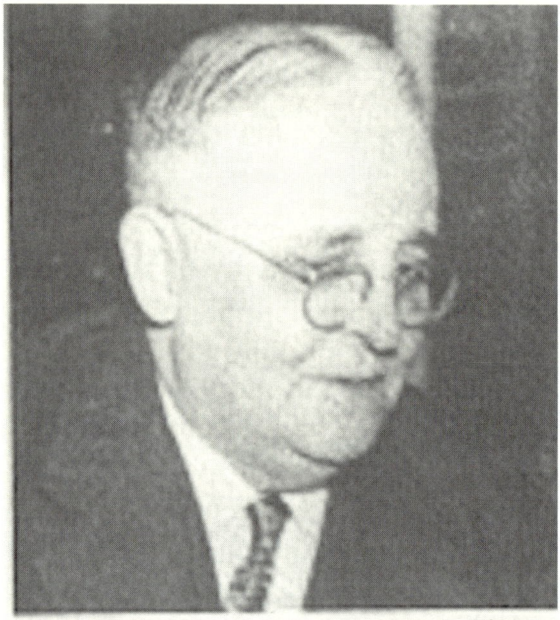

Superintendent Max Bahr

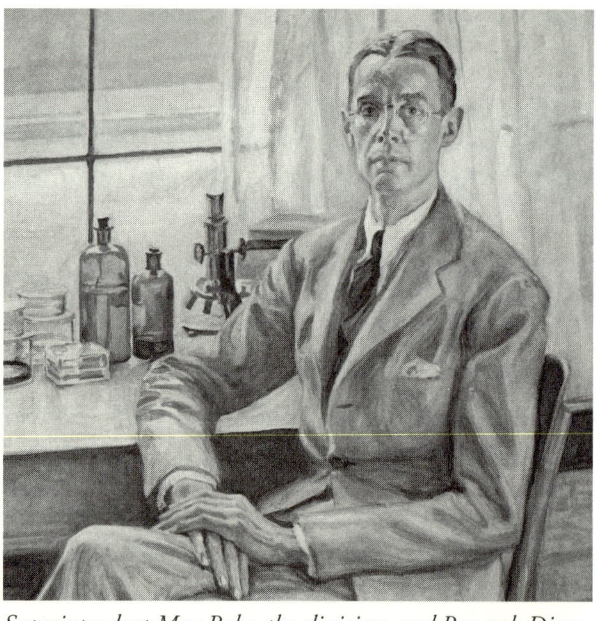

Superintendent Max Bahr, the clinician, and Research Director Walter Breutsch, the neuropathologist, met every Saturday morning at the Pathological Department to discuss and plan studies of new treatments for psychiatric disorders. Portrait by Indiana artist Ruth Pratt Bobbs.

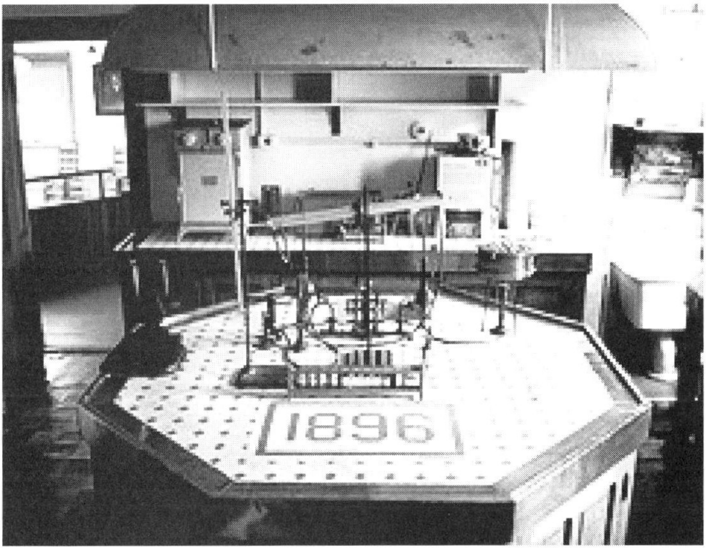

A laboratory in the Pathological Department, where chemical assays of components of body fluids and microscopic examination of blood cells were carried out. Many of the procedures performed here remained in common use in hospitals until mid-twentieth century.

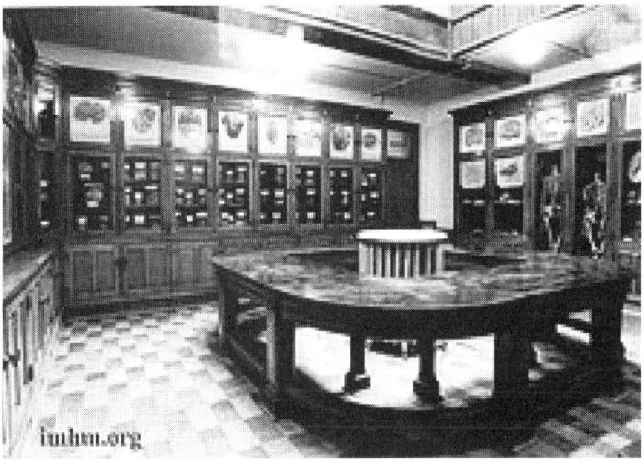

The circular oak table had space in the center for a professor to stand and demonstrate pathologic specimens from autopsies to students gathered in a circle around the outside of the table. The glass front cases lining the walls hold preserved specimens. These specimens are still there today in the Indiana Medical History Museum.

3
A Parallel Saga of State and Private Cooperation

Larue Carter Hospital I

In the last decades of the nineteenth century, even as Edenharter's Pathological Department was developed, Central State Hospital proved too small to care for all citizens of the state in need of psychiatric treatment. Other hospitals were gradually added to the system. Logansport State Hospital was opened in 1888 on the bluffs of Wabash River. Popularly known as "Longcliff" for this stunning location, it was created to serve those with mental illness living in the twenty-four counties in the northwest corridor of Indiana. The year 1890 saw two state hospitals added to Indiana's state hospital system. Evansville State Hospital, named "Woodmere," provided solitude and peace for mentally ill patients from the southwestern portion of Indiana, and Richmond State Hospital was opened to serve patients from the state's east central counties. Madison State Hospital, known as "Cragmont," was established in 1910 to serve southeastern Indiana. The hospital was designed in the "cottage" style of state hospital construction, with twenty two-story cottages that provided patients with maximum exposure to fresh air and natural light.

All of these facilities remain operational today. Logansport houses a special program for court-referred patients known as the Isaac Ray Unit, and Richmond contains the state hospital system's program for patients with a "dual diagnosis" of substance dependence and mental illness. They were joined in 1966 by a special state program for children ages 7 to 13, the Evansville Psychiatric Children's Center.[1]

The 1945 facility, Norman M. Beatty Hospital for the Criminally Insane, opened in Westville to house patients from Alaska with criminal histories. An arrangement approved by the state largely for financial reasons, the facility also held similar patients from within Indiana. The Indiana General Assembly turned the facility over to the Indiana Department of Corrections in 1977 as Westville Correctional Center.

The new Larue D. Carter Memorial Hospital established in the 1950s represented a gradual nationwide change from large state psychiatric hospitals housing several thousand patients to smaller facilities. Opening in 1952 on the campus of the School of Medicine in Indianapolis, its mission was to treat acutely ill patients, to teach medical students and residents, and to research treatments in psychiatry. In contrast to Central State Hospital for the Insane, which had housed well over two thousand patients at peak census, Larue Carter Hospital initially had a total of 250 beds with separate departments for children, adolescents, and adults. It would serve the state well in the next decades.

The story of this new version of Edenharter's dream began in Cincinnati in 1866 with the birth of Albert Eugene Sterne. Sterne was a good student who received his bachelor's degree from Harvard and then traveled to Europe, the Mecca of the day for medical training. While attaining his medical degree from the University of Berlin in 1891, he developed an interest in neuropsychiatry. Returning to the United States, he moved to Indianapolis, where he opened Norways Sanitarium, a private psychiatric hospital that would be part of the evolution of Larue Carter. He also joined the faculty of the Central Indiana College of Medicine and Surgery, one of the proprietary medical schools in Indiana at the time, as professor of neurology and psychiatry. Sterne's writings and commentary can be found in various proceedings of regional medical societies, as well as in the *Journal of the American Medical Association* and the *Journal of Nervous and Mental Diseases* from the turn of the twentieth century. He wrote a national journal article approving the imminent opening of Edenharter's "New Pathologic Institute of the Central State Hospital for the Insane" in 1897.[2]

The Norways Sanitarium was very successful, and Sterne became an influential figure in midwestern medical circles. He died suddenly at age 65 following the 1931 meeting of the American Medical Association, [3] and Larue Depew Carter, MD, assumed the directorship of Norways. A native Hoosier, born in Westfield in 1880, and a graduate of the Medical College of Indiana, Carter could easily speak the language of the state's politicians. Even though he had received additional medical training in Philadelphia, New York, and Baltimore, it did not diminish his local political influence that he had done his internship at the Indianapolis City Hospital and residency training in psychiatry and neurology at the Eastern Indiana Hospital for the Insane in Richmond. Articles about Carter at the time generally referred to him as "the dean of Indiana Neuropsychiatry."[4] His official title was Professor of Neurology in the Indiana University School of Medicine's neuropsychiatry department. Several other private psychiatrists in the community worked with Carter in his quest for improved psychiatric care and education in Indiana, including Philip Reed, MD, a later director of Norways Sanitarium; Earl Mericle, MD; John Greist, MD; and Keith Hepburn, MD.

From his prominent position as director of Norways, Carter began lobbying actively for a new central facility not only for the training of psychiatric residents, but also for all of the other mental health disciplines—nursing, psychology, social work, and occupational, physical, and recreational therapies. He was appointed the first president of the newly formed Indiana Mental Health Council, created to study treatment of mental illness in Indiana and to recommend and oversee mechanisms to improve it. This appointment put him in an even better position to work toward change. He spoke regularly before members of the Indiana General Assembly, urging them to pass legislation for the betterment of mental health. His focus was what Edenharter had initiated: the threefold mission of humane, science-based care of patients, education of physicians, and research on treatments of psychiatric disorders. In 1944 the General Assembly responded with an act calling for the creation of "a hospital . . . for instruction and research in mental illness under the supervision of the faculty of the Indiana University College of Medicine." Carter died on January 22, 1946, at his home in Indianapolis after several weeks of illness, two years prior to the 1948 groundbreaking for the new hospital.[5] Because of his tireless work on behalf of those with psychiatric illnesses, the hospital was named in Carter's memory.

Meanwhile David Boyd, MD, had been recruited in 1938 as chair of the developing academic department of psychiatry at Indiana University. Boyd had a national reputation for his long-time service as secretary to the American Board of Psychiatry and Neurology. Many consider him to have been the first official academic chairman of the Indiana University School of Medicine Department of Neuropsychiatry. Shortly after his arrival, the IU psychiatric residency training program was officially approved.

Boyd organized a teaching service within the City Hospital psychiatric program and instituted resident rotations there. This facility was later known as Marion County General Hospital and eventually as William Niles Wishard Memorial Hospital. In 1939 he began adding specific experiences with induction of convulsions with insulin and later electrical current, both then beginning to come into wide usage in the United States. Convulsive treatments were being used and studied concurrently by Bahr and Bruetsch at Central Indiana Hospital. The treatments were both part of education of medical students and psychiatry residents on clinical rotations at Norways Sanitarium.

With the onset of World War II, most of the psychiatrists in the community shipped overseas in military service. Teaching fell entirely on the shoulders of Boyd. By 1947, he had implemented a psychiatric curriculum for the junior year of medical school with assistance from Louis W. Nie, MD, who had received both bachelor and medical degrees from Indiana University and had served for a time on the faculty of the Department of Psychiatry. However, in 1948, Boyd took the senior position in the psychiatry department of the Mayo Clinic at Rochester, Minnesota, and Nie went into private practice with John Greist. With the loss of both Boyd and Nie, Alexander Ross, MD, became interim chairman of both neurology and psychiatry.

Finally in 1952, Herbert Gaskill, MD, was recruited from Philadelphia to chair psychiatry, with his younger colleague Philip Seitz, MD. They introduced psychoanalytic theory and practice into the department. Gaskill initiated a psychosomatic study group with collaboration from Lucia Tower, MD, of the Chicago Psychoanalytic Institute, and they had an impact on many of the area's psychiatric practitioners. But Gaskill left the department after only a year, recruited to the University of Colorado's Department of Psychiatry in Denver. During the search for a replacement chairman, Alexander Ross, MD, chairman of the Department of Neurology and chair of the search committee for the new psychiatry chairman, once again assumed interim administrative responsibilities and some limited teaching commitments in psychiatry. Ross was seen as an excellent clinician with "marvelous diagnostic acumen" and was a "magnificent teacher."[6] After considerable work to recruit an appropriate chair, Ross's search committee recommended John I. Nurnberger, Sr., MD, for the position.[7] Ross was impressed that Nurnberger had credentials in both neurology and psychiatry.

Meanwhile Juul C. Nielsen, MD, had become the first superintendent of Larue Carter Hospital in 1951. The superintendent of a state hospital, associated with a university medical center, is responsible not only for seeing that patients receive the best, most up-to-date care but also for hiring professionals and supervising education of trainees in psychiatry, psychology, nursing, social work, occupational therapy, and all the other disciplines that staff a modern psychiatric facility. In addition, clinical research facilities and researchers come under the purview of a superintendent. Electroconvulsive and other convulsive treatments (e.g., induced by medications such as insulin or metrazol) existed for mood disorders in the 1930s and 1940s, but in the 1950s the first new medications for psychiatric disorders became available and many newer approaches to psychotherapy, especially those of shorter term and of more focus on daily life, were being promoted. The training of psychiatry residents now included supervision in both, using a variety of psychotherapies and prescribing the new medications coming on the market. In addition, residents were exposed to research findings about all these new treatments and some had opportunity to do research themselves, working with experienced faculty as they carried out projects.

Nielsen was born on a farm in Denmark in 1896. Emigrating to the U.S. in 1914, he took work on a farm in Nebraska and became a naturalized citizen. He enlisted in the Army in 1917 and served as a medic during World War I, which convinced him to enter a career in medicine rather than farming. Returning to Nebraska after the war, he improved his English skills at Dana College in Blair, Nebraska, then earned his BS degree from the University of Nebraska in 1925. He worked his way through medical school there and interned at Emmanuel Hospital in Omaha.

His medical career began as he performed physical exams for the Union Pacific Railroad. Subsequently he entered general practice in Acadia, Nebraska. Not satisfied with general medicine, he did postgraduate work at the University of Colorado Psychopathic Hospital in 1930 and became superintendent of Norfolk (Nebraska) Hospital for the Insane in 1931. His next position was as superintendent and clinical director at Hastings State Hospital from 1933 to 1942. During this time, Nielsen did research on treatment of general paresis with the use of fever induction, as had Bahr and Bruetsch at Central State, and on convulsive therapy.[8] He became certified by the American Board of Psychiatry and Neurology in 1938. Enlisting in the army again in World War II, he was commissioned as a major in the Medical Corps and worked on psychiatric approaches to better treat soldiers for "battle fatigue," as PTSD was then known. Returning to Hastings in 1945, he was again superintendent there until coming to Larue D. Carter Memorial Hospital as its inaugural superintendent in 1951.[9]

Nielsen was one of the country's foremost neuropsychiatrists at the time of his recruitment to Carter, recommended as one of the "outstanding state hospital men in the country."[10] He was a counselor of the American Psychiatric Association and was known as an expert in the treatments of the day, including fever treatments for paresis and also electroconvulsive, metrazol, and insulin coma therapies for schizophrenia and mood disorders. He would become the first president of the Society of Biological Psychiatry. Chosen at Carter Hospital for both his administrative abilities and his keen eye for staff recruitment, he was brought in as the first employee of the hospital in 1951 so that he could build the new hospital's staff from scratch before the hospital was to open in 1952.

Larue Carter Hospital had been envisioned as a new facility built upon new philosophies and scientifically proven treatment techniques. Nielsen described these in an article in *The Modern Hospital* in March 1954. The purposes of Carter Hospital, built at a cost of $4,650,000, would be to provide intensive care to treat psychiatric disorders quickly and to train all staff in administering such care. Rapid recovery and return to the community would replace lengthy custodial care. The entire structure of the building focused on these goals. Two V-shaped wings for patient wards extended from a central unit. The wings provided light and ventilation for patients as well as privacy because other patients couldn't look into their windows. The color scheme used pastel tints. Each patient had a comfortable, upholstered easy chair. Each ward had a living room with comfortable furniture, puzzles, games, and ping-pong equipment. Food, planned by nutritionists, was served on each unit cafeteria style so that patients would have some choice. The hospital had a patients' library with a variety of materials to serve many interests, beauty and barber shops, and a snack bar. Patients spent from two to four hours daily in occupational therapy that included creative, industrial, musical, and domestic arts. Recreational activities were held six nights a week. A psychology department provided diagnostic services, education, and research in providing psychological testing to better understand patients' behavior.

But then, as has often been true, plans for better treatment of the mentally ill foundered on the rocks of funding. Nielsen was almost immediately embroiled in political controversy, criticized by the leadership in county and city government for not staffing the hospital and filling it with patients quickly enough, and by state policy makers for wanting to spend too much money to acquire the kind of staff he felt were necessary.[11] At one point, the mayor of Indianapolis proposed transferring individuals from the city jail to the unused beds at Larue Carter Hospital. Commissioner of Mental Health Margaret Morgan, MD, like Edenharter, Bahr, and Carter a politically savvy physician, instead transferred psychiatric patients from the Marion County General Hospital to Carter Hospital and psychiatrically ill inmates at the city jail to a locked ward at the General Hospital. Once again a progressive physician had kept patient care on a medical basis rather than subject to the vagaries of politics. Her decision had also filled some of the empty beds at Larue Carter Hospital.

Underlying these other problems was the salary structure for staff at Carter Hospital. Nielsen was caught in a "Catch 22": in order to admit more patients, he needed more staff; in order to obtain more staff, he needed better funding; and in order to have more funds, he needed to admit more patients. The state budget committee finally increased salaries for Larue Carter Hospital staff in 1953.[12]

Commissioner Morgan had many other political battles and was simultaneously trying to fund a new Institute of Psychiatric Research as a companion facility for Carter Hospital, replacing the aging Pathological Department at Central State Hospital. She could not always be the ally that Nielsen needed to fulfill his vision at Carter Hospital.[13] Nielsen resigned as superintendent in 1955, moving on to the superintendent's job at Central State Hospital in Petersburg, Virginia, and then returning for one final tour of duty as superintendent at Hastings State Hospital prior to his retirement to Naples, Florida, in 1962. There, Dr. Nielsen and his daughter, Polly, helped to establish a mental health center, the latest system for modern treatment of the mentally ill.[14] He died in Florida in 1970 at the age of 74.

Notes

1. Historic Asylums of America, http://www.rootsweb.ancestry.com/~asylums/.
2. A. E. Sterne, "The New Pathological Institute of the Central Indiana Hospital for the Insane," *Journal of Nervous and Mental Disease* 24 (1897): 58–61.
3. Obituary column, *Journal of Nervous and Mental Disease* 74 (1931): 785.
4. *The Courier*, Nov. 6, No. 8, May 20, 1958.
5. *Indiana Biography* 29: 116; IR 920 13856.
6 C. Bonsett, Indiana Medicine Oral History Project, Box 1, Folder 7, W. H. Smith Library, Indiana Historical Society, Indianapolis.
7. Adapted from a brief reminiscence on the history of the Indiana University Department of Psychiatry, Dr. John I. Nurnberger, Sr., 1980.
8. J. C. Nielsen, J. R. Marx, and H. A. Dickel, "Artificial Fever Therapy in Juvenile Neurosyphilis," *Archives of Dermatology* 45 (1942): 688–93.
9. Unpublished biographical correspondence from Dr. Nielsen's children, Juul C. Nielsen, Jr., and Polly Keller.
10. "Dr. Juul C. Nielsen to Head New Carter Mental Hospital," *Indianapolis Star*, March 25, 1951.
11. "Idle Carter Hospital Beds Draw Clark Fire," *Indianapolis Star*, July 21, 1953.
12. "Mental Hospital to Open New Space" by Jack Averitt, *Indianapolis News*, August 8, 1953.
13. "Judge Praises Nielsen Role at Larue Carter," *Indianapolis Times*, September 6, 1956.
14. Classified Advertising: "Naples on the Gulf MHC," *Community Mental Health Journal* 5 (1969): 193.

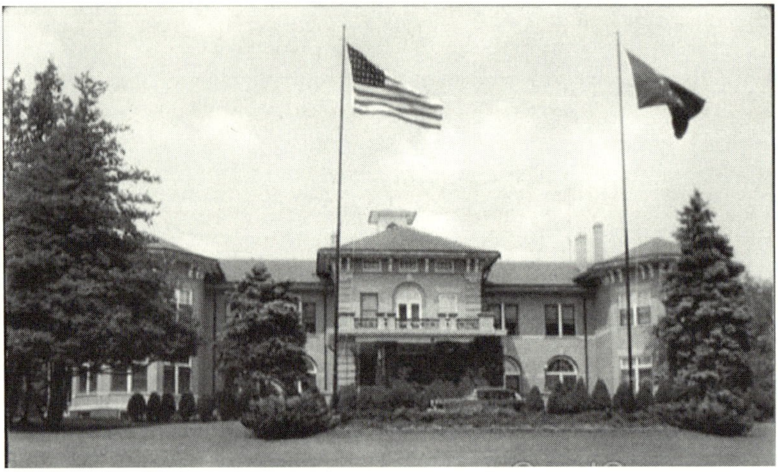

Southeastern Indiana Hospital in Madison, "Cragmont," overlooking the Ohio River, opened in 1910. It is near Clifty Falls State Park and is considered the most beautiful location of any of the state hospitals.

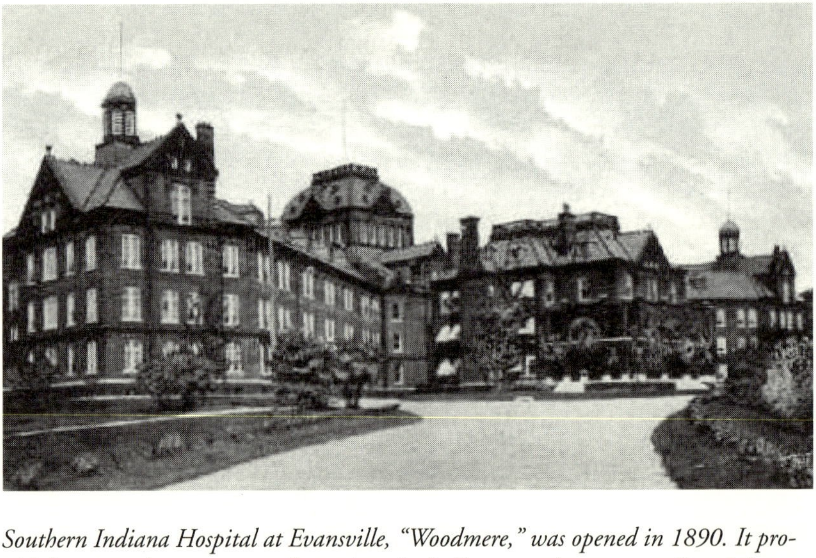

Southern Indiana Hospital at Evansville, "Woodmere," was opened in 1890. It provided many unique programs for patients including an orchestra, a reading club, a Toastmaster's club, and a homemaker's club.

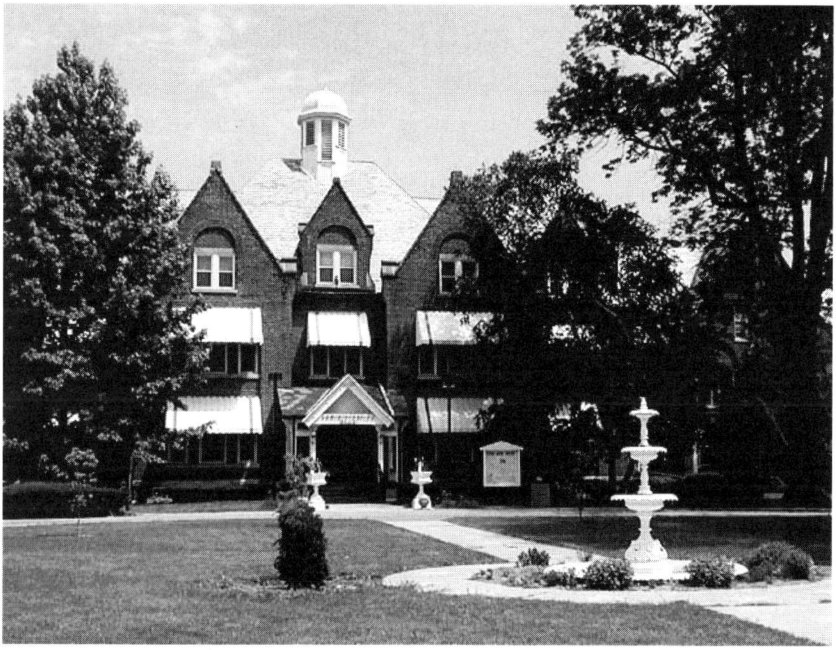

Eastern Indiana Hospital at Richmond, "Easthaven," was opened in 1890 in renovated buildings that had housed mentally disabled individuals (called "feeble-minded" at the time). In the early days, when it was time for meals and other scheduled events patients were summoned by a steam whistle.

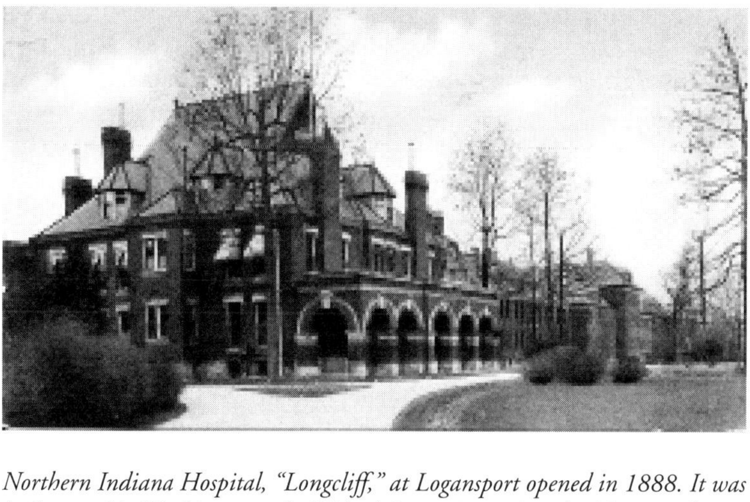

Northern Indiana Hospital, "Longcliff," at Logansport opened in 1888. It was built on a bluff looking over the Wabash River. By 1940 it had become the largest state psychiatric hospital with 2,383 beds.

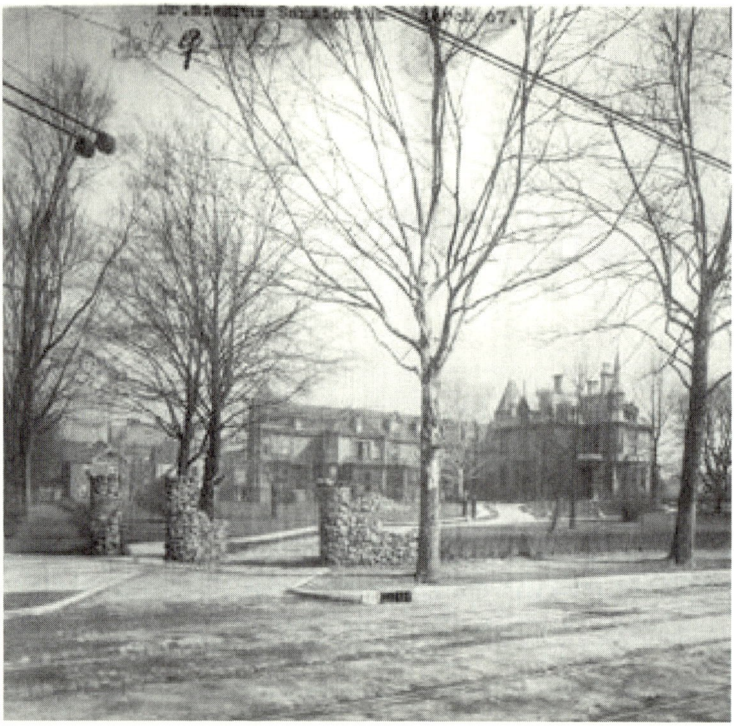

Norways Sanitarium was the second private psychiatric hospital in Indianapolis, founded in 1898, ten years after the first, Neuronhurst. Norways outlasted Neuronhurst by twenty years, closing in 1957 on the east side of Indianapolis. Norways had a psychiatry residency program and received grant money when more became available for psychiatry in the 1950s. Information about hospitals is from P. M. Coons and E. S. Bowman, Psychiatry in Indiana: The First 175 Years (*Bloomington IN: IUniverse, Inc., 2010).*

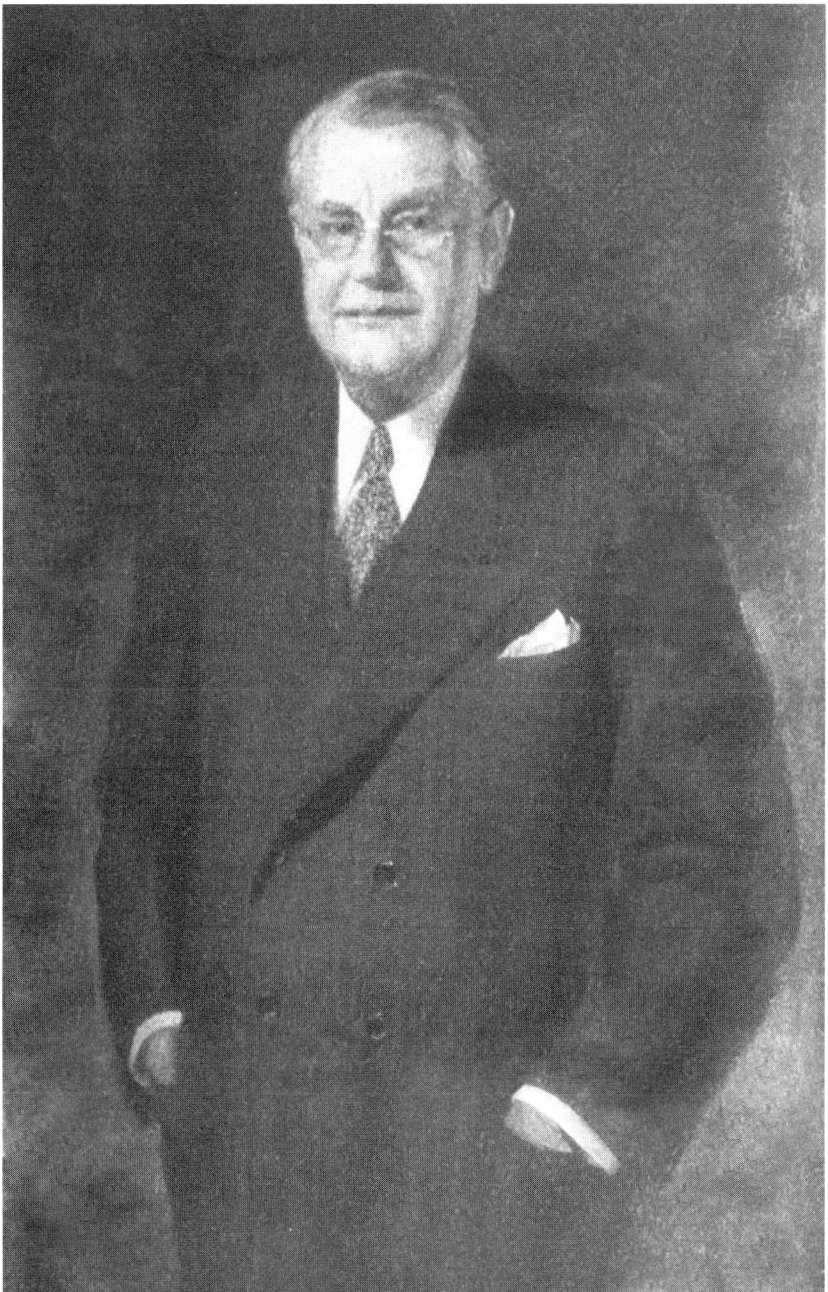

Dr. Larue Carter (1880–1946) joined the faculty of Indiana University School of Medicine in 1914. Except for service in the Medical Corps in World War I, he remained on the faculty until his death. Portrait by Indiana artist Wayman Adams..

4
Exploring With Unrelenting Enthusiasm

The Institute of Psychiatric Research I

The building of the Institute of Psychiatric Research had been spearheaded by Margaret Morgan, Indiana's first commissioner of mental health. After three years on the faculty of the department of psychiatry at the medical school, she was appointed commissioner by the newly elected governor, George N. Craig, who had run on a campaign that promised improvement of state mental institutions.[1] The Pathological Department at Central was no longer what it had been. Some other, new research and teaching facility was needed. That new facility would be part of a forward-thinking approach to mental health in the state, one based on rapid treatment in improved facilities with a strong focus on research that would necessitate an adequate building.

Morgan and Governor Craig's work in convincing the state legislature to devote more funds to psychiatric treatment was lauded nationally by *Time* magazine.[2] Pointing out that acute treatment would shorten hospital stays, Morgan convinced the legislators that hiring more doctors, nurses, and other personnel for state hospitals would save money in the long run. If patients were actively treated early in the course of their illnesses, they would be less likely to need long-term care in state hospitals. She also pointed out that research would provide prevention and cure for mental illnesses, thus diminishing the need for state hospital beds. Her observation was prescient. State hospital populations declined in the 1960s with the availability of new medications for psychiatric treatment, many of them studied at Larue Carter Hospital and the Institute of Psychiatric Research.

The institute was dedicated December 13, 1956, almost sixty years to the day after the dedication of the Pathological Department. Times had changed, especially in psychiatry. The institute was a $1,500,000, four-story, 50,000-square-foot building containing laboratory and office space, a large conference/seminar room, and additional support areas including a cold room, glassware room, mechanical and electronic shops, a loading dock, and utility areas. Money allocated by the legislature to the Department of Mental Health had built the building, but the research would be funded by both public and private funds.[3] Federal funds were becoming available through the National Institute of Mental Health at the National Institutes of Health, and various private foundations were funding more mental health research. Daniel Blain, MD, medical director of the American Psychiatric Association, spoke at the ceremony, pointing out that Indiana had risen from fortieth to sixth among the states in mental health programs. "Whatever the years ahead may hold for the mentally ill," he said, "among the beacon lights to comfort them will be this splendid Psychiatric Research Institute facility."

Commissioner Morgan observed, "We have been fortunate to obtain some of the most outstanding professional and business people in the country to serve as members of the board of directors. The Institute which we dedicate today stands as a symbol of hope for the future. I am pleased that we have been able to establish this institute which will remind us of new frontiers to be opened up through research."[4] The original board of directors for the institute recruited by Dr. Morgan included Herman Wells, president of Indiana University; John Van Nuys, dean of the medical school; Mrs. Albert Lasker, president of the Lasker Foundation; Homer Hargrave, director of the Chicago Association of Commerce and Industry; James Adams of the board of directors of Libby-Owens-Ford Glass Company; Mrs. Oscar Ahlgren, assistant to the director of the U.S. Treasury Department Savings Bond Division; and J. Irwin Miller, chairman of the board of Cummins Engine Company and Irwin Union Bank and Trust of Columbus, Indiana.[5]

John I. Nurnberger, Sr., MD, the new director, had impeccable credentials and experience. Both public and press expected him to be a fine director of the new facility. Nurnberger was a pioneer in American psychiatry in his day, just as Edenharter had been sixty years earlier. In 1956, when Nurnberger came to Indiana University School of Medicine as chairman of the department of psychiatry, he also became director of the new Institute of Psychiatric Research and prepared to direct affairs at this state-of-the-art laboratory building to study neurobiology related to behavior and to psychiatric disorders. He had credentials and experience in psychiatry, neurology, and histology (microscopic cell structure) and had held teaching and research positions at the Institute of Living in Hartford, Connecticut, and at Yale University Department of Neurology and Psychiatry. In describing his philosophy in setting up the institute, Nurnberger wrote:

> In no branch of medical sciences is knowledge about the origins and treatment of human disorders so incomplete and inadequate as it is in psychiatry. This is entirely understandable when one appreciates the widespread ramifications of emotional and mental disturbance. These touch every aspect of emotional life and mental activity and are likewise reflected in myriad ways in intimate machinery of bodily action and organ functions. A medical discipline such as psychiatry whose domain includes significant factors influencing the development of the human individual before birth as well as those genetic, physical, psychic and emotional factors which underlie normal growth and development must of necessity evolve slowly . . . [and] must be explored with unrelenting enthusiasm by the most sensitive and discriminating scientific methods in the hands of the most gifted and dedicated research investigators possible in any field.

He went on to write in his *First Annual Report*: "However intangible may be the disturbed thoughts, feelings, motivations, or urges which are the province of psychiatry, there can be no question that the poignant distress and anguish of the mentally and emotionally disturbed and of their affected relatives and friends are real and urgent." This view led Nurnberger to explore those intangibles with "unrelenting enthusiasm." But he was realistic. As he and his colleagues set about on their scientific explorations, he realized that ". . . we are still largely in ignorance of the necessary or even significant contributory causes of the major mental and emotional disorders of man. Our most useful treatment procedures, whether physical, social, or psychological, are still very largely 'trial and error' instruments, and the actual results achieved are just now coming under critical scrutiny."[6] As with any other research—especially because they were using newly developed methods of others and developing methods of their own—the scientists at the Institute of Psychiatric Research knew there would be false leads and setbacks as well as the enthusiastically-hoped-for breakthroughs. These concerns were especially important for studying the human brain in an ethical manner, necessitating indirect studies of blood, urine, spinal fluid, and the like. Through the coming decades there would be increasingly sophisticated methods of studying the brain, culminating in noninvasive neuroimaging techniques ("X-rays" and other methods of visualizing the brain in living individuals) that posed no danger to patients.

Nurnberger assembled for the institute a multidisciplinary team by recruitment from other universities as well as from departments of Indiana University. They included biochemists, behavioral psychologists, and psychiatric and neurologic clinicians who would study what was happening in the brain during behavioral changes and psychiatric disorders. They worked with Donald Moore, MD, who was superintendent of Larue Carter Hospital when Nurnberger came to Indianapolis, and his staff studying patients at Carter Hospital as well as doing research with laboratory animals at the Institute of Psychiatric Research. The institute was located on the medical school campus across the street from Larue Carter Hospital, the other institution fulfilling Edenharter's dream. An underground tunnel even connected the two buildings. All members of the research staff taught medical students, residents in psychiatry, graduate students (especially in neurochemistry), and fellows in various areas of psychiatry and neurology. Medical students were able to spend time participating in research at the institute. Staff published papers and presented data at national scientific meetings, served on university and national committees, and indirectly helped attract physicians to the medical school and throughout the state.

In the absence of modern techniques to study brain chemistry, American psychiatrists in the first half of the twentieth century had focused on psychological treatments and theories, especially the psychoanalytic techniques of Sigmund Freud and his contemporaries. By no means discounting psychological treatment, Nurnberger was one of the few psychiatry department chairmen in the United States at the time—mostly in the Midwest, e.g., Paul Huston, MD, at the University of Iowa and Edwin Gildea, MD, at Washington University in St. Louis—who also saw the importance of biological studies. The research initiated by these visionaries would end arguments about whether "nature" (biology) or "nurture" (social environment) is important in determining normal behavior as well as psychiatric illness. Both are important, and they are related and complementary, a fact that would soon be demonstrated at the institute by Morris Aprison, PhD. Nurnberger's broad perspective is reflected in a textbook for medical students that he coauthored. The book included sections on the biologic substrata of behavior, the psychosocial determinants of behavior, and the essentials of a science of behavior.[7]

Research in psychiatry was moving from outward observations of behavior to observation of the workings of the brain itself and, ultimately, to a correlation of findings from both kinds of observations in order to understand the entire system of brain and behavior. During the first year, Nurnberger was busy recruiting staff and equipping the new laboratories. He designed a pharmacologic research project at Central State Hospital and organized a committee with other medical faculty, including Dean Van Nuys, to study biological growth and development. Psychologist Eugene Levitt, PhD, and biochemist Harold Persky, PhD, of the new institute staff initiated research about psychological and metabolic aspects of normal pregnancy and labor and the impact of sociocultural factors on infant and child development in collaboration with the Department of Obstetrics and Gynecology and the Department of Pediatrics. Persky, who had come from the University of Chicago, also studied correlates of stress hormones and anxiety. Biochemist Aprison was recruited from Galesburg State Research Hospital in Illinois. Aprison would direct groundbreaking studies of neurotransmitters, the chemical messengers in the brain, and their correlations with behavior in animals. He investigated chemical substances in blood and urine of schizophrenic patients and normal human subjects with senior research fellow Hanus J. Grosz, MD; Richard E. McCaman, PhD, recruited from Washington University in St. Louis, developed microassays of biochemical components of extremely small bits of brain tissue.[8]

Neurologist Arthur L. Drew, MD, acting associate director of the institute, investigated the biochemical genetics of neurological diseases, setting up collaboration with the Department of Pediatrics for clinical research and treatment. Psychologist Marvin Zuckerman, PhD, and Grosz studied attitudes of parents of schizophrenic patients at Larue Carter Hospital and parents of normal individuals. This was important research because it was still thought by many at the time that parenting practices caused schizophrenia, which turned out not to be the case. Zuckerman implemented preliminary research that would lead to multidisciplinary studies of psychological, behavioral, and perceptual distortions in acutely developing schizophrenia in hospitalized patients, of value in differentiating this serious disorder as early as it could be done in order to begin treatment as soon as possible.[9] Work continues to this day at the Prevention and Recovery Center for Schizophrenia in the Department of Psychiatry under the direction of Alan Breier, MD.

Charles B. Ferster, PhD, who had collaborated with well-known behavioral psychologist B. F. Skinner, PhD, developed operant conditioning equipment for studying behavior in laboratory animals, manipulating rewards and aversive events to maintain complex forms of behavior. Harvard L. Armus, PhD, studied problems of motivation using new techniques for continuously recording behavior of laboratory animals and was able to elaborate findings about motivational aspects of conflict and to quantify the effects of various schedules of rewards on motivation.[10]

After the initial year of setting up research laboratories at the institute, the first full year of uninterrupted work by the staff, 1958, saw a "solid core of . . . mental health scientists, representing many different disciplines and varied professional training" acquire "a sense of collective identity and collaborative enthusiasm." Each investigator "was encouraged to pursue his own investigative interests and in his own way."[11] Nurnberger noted at the time:

> . . . such an organization is rather unusual in the field of mental health research. For the past seventy years or more the talents of many clinical and laboratory scientists have been focused on major problems in mental health and disease. Millions of words have been published on the origins, nature, and management of psychotic and neurotic disturbances, on mental deficiency, on the structure and function of the ordered and disordered human brain, on the baffling interrelations between mind and body, feelings and thoughts, impulse and act. . . . The majority of past work has been topically oriented and paternalistically directed. Out of such activities have come our usual multi- or interdisciplinary research programs. Centrally coordinated groups have on occasion, been formed specifically to investigate schizophrenia, retraining and reeducation of the retarded, problems of aging, the role of anxiety in emotional disorders, the neural mechanisms of conditioned behavior, to mention but a few. Intensive focusing of the activities of many workers has been implemented in this way. There is no question that research, so organized, has provided much useful information and has expanded available knowledge. In spite of such long term investigative work we are still largely in ignorance of the necessary or even significant contributory causes of the major mental and emotional disorders of man. . . . It is evident that major advances presume a fresh and unpreju-

> diced look, and very likely from new and even unfamiliar vantage points. Centrally coordinated research activity of topical orientation has suffered from the serious limitation of casting inquiry in conventional moulds. The authoritarian organization of many research groups has tended, albeit unwittingly, to submerge original inquiry and the unusual point of view in a maze of organizational or committee protocol. It is for these reasons that a serious and continued effort has been expended to encourage independently conceived and conducted research in the Institute.[12]

This approach would include both basic and applied research focused on quality rather than on total number of publications.[13] Publications did come about, reaching more than fifty annually in the first few years, by staff members who also had administrative, teaching, and clinical duties. The institute's tone was set so that each investigator would pursue his or her own research interests rather than setting out specifically to discover the cause and cure of a specific disorder. For example, rather than looking for the causes and cure of schizophrenia, researchers would study brain chemistry and then observe how it might be disturbed in patients with schizophrenia. This approach has subsequently been demonstrated to make discoveries related to causes and cures and to pave the way for better understanding of psychiatric disorders. Psychologist Joseph Hingtgen, PhD, recalls:

> The excitement of the [institute] atmosphere was contagious. Medical students from the late 1950s still remember a most impressive lecture when a faculty member from the Institute brought a pigeon in a box to class, and showed how it responded to colored discs that brought a reward, but stopped working for non-rewarded colored discs. Other medical students at that time were intrigued by the innovative concept of brain chemistry being directly correlated with behavior. The Institute was considered one of the major early centers for biological psychiatry research in the USA.[14]

Nurnberger not only had brought together a group of scientists and clinicians from many disciplines, but also had given them academic freedom to pursue their own interests, and this policy worked. Scientists from many disciplines gathered in the same institute, exchanging views, presenting reviews of their own research, and interacting with scientists from around the world who were invited to give seminars to faculty and students. Dr. Hingtgen recalls that "Institute faculty lunch hours were scenes of emotionally heated scientific exchanges, which often went on with no set time limit."[15] Open exchanges of views among institute staff—active, intelligent, creative individuals formulating different hypotheses in the newly developing field of neurobiology—inevitably led to personality clashes. In this "exciting and productive atmosphere," Nurnberger was a "wonderful peacemaker," very good at settling disputes when egos got out of hand.[16] He believed that "interdisciplinary research based on *questions to be answered rather than an administrative edict*" would "bear special fruit in encouraging new and unusual approaches to the mental health problems we face" [emphasis added].[17] For example, in line with Nurnberger's idea of collaboration by experts using the expertise of each, Aprison and Ferster expanded their research correlating brain neurotransmitter changes with behavioral changes in laboratory animals, being among the first researchers to do so.

Neurons, Neurotransmiters, and Synapses. . .

The basic functions of the nervous system are carried out by transmission of electrical currents along nerve cells (neurons) and their appendages, incoming projections of the cell body (dendrites) and outgoing fibers (axons) that will join those from other cells to form nerves. Currents are generated by the passage of electrolytes like sodium and potassium ions back and forth across the membranes that envelop neurons, dendrites, and axons. The space between two neurons (axon of one, dendrite or cell body of the other) is called a synapse. At the end of a presynaptic axon, a neurotransmitter such as serotonin, norepinephrine, dopamine, glutamate, GABA, or acetylcholine is released into the synapse to attach to receptors on the postsynaptic neuron and, through a series of chemical reactions, stimulate electrical current flow in that neuron. Some of these neurotransmitters had been studied in the nerves of the body for decades.

By the 1950s it was becoming understood that they were important in the brain as well and might be related to causes and treatments of psychiatric disorders. Studying the chemistry of the brain was much more difficult than studying nerves in the body. The chemistry of human brains had been measured at autopsy, but chemical changes would already have occurred with death. Research on brains of laboratory animals had been done, but again the techniques themselves tended to alter the very chemical reactions to be studied. New methods were becoming available.

[See illustration p. 72.]]

Studies on neurotransmitters and the chemical reactions that synthesized and metabolized them were being developed internationally. It still wasn't clear which chemicals were important neurotransmitters in the central nervous system—brain and spinal cord—or just how they were related to behavior or to psychiatric disorders. At the cutting edge of contemporary science, Aprison and Ferster began research on serotonin, at the time proposed as an important neurotransmitter in the brain possibly related to depression. In the brain, serotonin and certain other neurotransmitters are destroyed by the enzyme monoamine oxidase after use. The first antidepressants, marketed in the 1950s, were monoamine oxidase inhibitors—that is, by blocking destruction of serotonin and other neurotransmitters, they increased the concentration in the brain of these neurotransmitters. Clinically, they improved major depression in patients. As always with translating laboratory animal data to clinical effects of medication, the question remained whether or not the laboratory finding of increasing levels of neurotransmitters was related to the clinical effect of improving severe depression—or were they just two separate and unrelated effects of the medication?

Although serotonin does not readily pass from the blood into brain tissue, its precursor does. Intramuscular administration of the precursor, 5-hydroxytryptophan (5-HTP), increases levels of serotonin in the brain. (The 5-HTP travels from the injection site through the blood stream to the brain, where it is converted to serotonin.) Administration of the monoamine oxidase inhibitor iproniazid also increases serotonin in the brain by blocking the breakdown of serotonin by monoamine oxidase. Iproniazid was the first antidepressant medication. Aprison and Ferster studied pigeons in the classic Skinner box in which birds peck at a disc to receive food. When 5-HTP was given, pigeons stopped pecking. There was a dose-response ratio—the higher the dose of 5-HTP, the longer the pause in pecking. Iproniazid also stopped the pecking. Giving both 5-HTP and iproniazid produced a greater effect than either alone.[18] Using several ways of manipulating brain serotonin, the researchers had demonstrated a correlation between brain serotonin level and a specific behavior, a breakthrough in understanding correlation of brain neurotransmitters and behavior and a demonstration of the interaction between brain biology and behavior in response to environment.

Ferster also examined the effects of sedative and stimulant drugs on conditioned behavior in laboratory animals. McCaman developed microtechniques to study brain enzymes, the effects of vitamins in the brain, and the chemistry of brain tumors in collaboration with researchers in the Department of Neurology. He later developed microassays for monoamine oxidase and other enzymes for Aprison's research, developing new methods applicable to very small amounts of tissue.[19]

Classical and Operant Conditioning of Behavior

"Classical" conditioning, originated by Ivan Pavlov in Russia, involves training a subject to respond to a neutral object in the same way as to an object that normally produces a certain response. For example, when a dog is presented with meat, it salivates. If a ticking noise sounds every time meat is presented, eventually the dog will salivate if the ticking noise sounds without meat being present. It has become "conditioned" to salivate when a ticking noise sounds, not a normal response.

In the "operant" conditioning of B. F. Skinner, an American who worked for a time at Indiana University in Bloomington, normal behaviors are "shaped" until a specific behavior occurs. For example, a pigeon is placed in a box with different colored discs. One disc, if pecked, will release grains of corn. The pigeon will normally peck randomly about the box. As it pecks different discs, it will eventually peck the one that rewards it with corn. Subsequently, when it is placed in the box, the pigeon will peck at the disc that produces the food reward. "Random" behaviors (pecking about the box) have been "shaped" to specific behavior (pecking only the disc that releases corn).

These and other behavioral conditioning strategies require multiple trials in the laboratory to achieve the desired change in behavior, a time-consuming process. Findings from laboratory animals can be applied to human behavior.

Persky and Levitt studied patients and normal subjects with regard to levels of anxiety and measured both psychological factors and blood levels of hormones related to stress—the adrenal hormone, hydrocortisone, and the pituitary hormone ACTH that directs production of hydrocortisone. They were looking at hypnotically induced anxiety and planning to study other emotions such as anger, depression, and the like. Later research in collaboration with the Department of Obstetrics and Gynecology expanded their studies from adrenal and pituitary hormones to female hormones. They developed new assays for measuring hormones. Several active medications were evaluated for effects on anxiety and hormones.[20]

Nurnberger, Levitt, and Zuckerman worked with the Department of Obstetrics and Gynecology in a pilot study of psychiatric, psychological, and endocrine factors in first pregnancies in young prenatal clinic patients. Nurnberger also collaborated with Theodore Tausig, MD, chief of neuropsychiatry at the veterans' hospital, to evaluate new admissions in order to appraise the role of sociocultural and economic factors in admission of patients to the psychiatry service. Later, Nurnberger, Zuckerman, and statistician James E. Norton made a sociocultural analysis of the ninety-two Indiana counties in relation to county utilization of state hospital facilities, information that would be invaluable for state planning for facilities.[21] In other words, they were considering family and environmental factors, not just diagnosis and severity of illness, that influence what a given patient will decide about hospitalization.

And so the work was well underway and prospering. During the second year, Drew, who had been in Japan, returned to become associate director of the institute. He was joined by Marilyn McCaman, who had just come on the staff after completing a PhD in pharmacology at Washington University in St. Louis. They continued Drew's previous research on muscular dystrophy. Another new staff scientist, John Paul Brady, MD, had completed his psychiatry residency at Institute of Living in Connecticut. Working with Ferster, he used operant conditioning techniques to study the behavior of patients and began work with Persky studying hormones in anxiety. He treated a patient with psychological blindness by use of operant conditioning to various objects in the environment, rewarding the patient each time she could identify an object and using objects that were increasingly difficult to see. The behavioral treatment ultimately cured the blindness.[22]

Later Brady worked with mathematician Claude J. Marmasse, DSc, developing mathematical models for predicting animal behavior in learning situations involving avoidance of unpleasant stimuli. Brady and Zuckerman studied effects of drugs on hypnotically induced emotional states, and Brady collaborated with Levitt to study psychological characteristics of human volunteers for behavioral experiments and with physiological psychologist Donald Doehring, PhD, to explore relationships between different kinds of conditioning and the accompanying physiologic responses to each.

After completing a PhD in social psychology at Michigan State University, Arturo DeHoyos joined the institute staff in 1961. He developed research questionnaires to study occupational and family stability, physical mobility, and social affiliation in patients and non-patient controls, especially in poor and minority communities. He began broader epidemiologic study of patterns of mental illness using records from the state Department of Mental Health.

In 1962 Nurnberger summarized the first five years of research at the institute.[22] Hormonal mechanisms of emotionality had been studied throughout the period by more than a dozen biochemists, psychologists, psychiatrists, mathematicians, and obstetricians and gynecologists. They brought expertise from their earlier research elsewhere on endocrine concomitants of anxiety and depression. He stated:

> Hypnotic techniques for generating clinically significant levels of anxiety in volunteer human subjects were perfected. Broad similarities in clinical symptomatology, biological concomitants and psychological performances were noted between such experimentally-induced arousal states and naturally-occurring psychiatric disturbances associated with increased anxiety levels. Under carefully-controlled conditions, the relationship between intensity of induced anxiety and nature and degree of activation of pituitary [and] adrenal cortical . . . mechanisms has been systematically explored. A significant role for pituitary adrenocorticotrophic [ACTH] mechanisms . . . had been defined. There appears to be a near-quantitative relation between magnitude of adrenal cortical activation and level of anxiety manifested. [23]

The institute would become known for studying models

of psychiatric disorders. Here, researchers developed a model of anxiety by discussing anxiety-producing situations with a hypnotized subject. The response of stress hormones in these subjects was the same as in individuals with anxiety disorders, i.e., the model seemed to mimic disorders. By making models of disorders with human volunteers or in laboratory animals and studying the various factors involved—which of those seem related to the disorder and which do not—researchers can better understand the disorder.

During the first five years (1957–1962) of the institute, two groups were working on basic biochemistry of the central nervous system. Both had worked with collaborators from biochemistry, neurology, neuropathology, pediatrics, neurosurgery, and psychiatry. A more detailed and specific description of their achievement follows:

> Aprison's group primarily focused on the dynamic neurohumoral [hormone effects on the brain] aspects of brain chemistry, the intra- and inter-species distribution characteristics of monoamine oxidase, serotonin, acetylcholine, and cholinesterase [an enzyme that breaks down acetylcholine] have been mapped for important nuclear masses [groups of neurons] and functionally distinct neural areas. Supporting data concerning the quantitative distribution of sodium, potassium, chloride, and water have been determined for the same nuclei areas. On an intracellular level, the particulate distribution of brain cholinesterase has been studied intensively, and major efforts have been made to lay the groundwork for the isolation, in pure molecular species of brain cholinesterase. Such an achievement would be of great importance, since it would make possible the physical and chemical characterization of the important enzyme or enzymes.

Meanwhile, the other group of neurochemists, working in McCaman's laboratory, was studying the chemistry of myelin, a lipid, or fatty substance that forms the protective sheath around nerve fibers. Transport across the myelin sheath is now known to be important in psychiatric disorders, especially mood disorders. McCaman's group was studying not only normal metabolism but also lipid metabolism in brain tumors. The combined research of Aprison and McCaman groups, Nurnberg's report concluded

> . . .*permitted a chemical "dissection"' of brain*, its important nuclear masses [small groups of neurons] and functionally distinct areas on *a level and with a degree of detail never before possible.*" [emphasis added] Not only an extended enzymatic mapping of brain parts, but also an expanding quantitative description of significant [chemical] concentrations is rapidly emerging, so that the time for a definitive synthesis of such important intra- and inter-species data is rapidly approaching. With such a rich background of normal information and with such a broad spectrum of microanalytic techniques it has been possible to conduct more extensive biochemical studies of human brain biopsies than previously thought possible. Biopsy studies of important central nervous system diseases encountered in childhood and adolescence are now in progress on a broad collaborative basis.

The latter included the work of Drew and McCaman.

In this *Fifth Annual Report*, Nurnberger also noted that studies begun with the Department of Obstetrics and Gynecology "provided interesting leads concerning the importance of prenatal maternal anxiety on the labor and delivery of a population of primigravida [first pregnancy] clinic patients. . . . the number and severity of physical complaints during pregnancy were closely related to the level of maternal anxiety" as was the amount of pain medication requested during the first stage of delivery. "Significant positive correlations between amount of neonatal motor activity and crying behavior and level of anxiety of the mother during her pregnancy have been discovered." These studies were continuing during the period, as was related research with the Department of Pediatrics about childrearing practices. These researches were being tied in with studies at Larue Carter Hospital about developmental history and determinants of disturbed behavior in autistic and schizophrenic children.

Scientists at the institute in this first five-year period carried out studies of human behavior in laboratory situations and changes with various new medications. They employed questionnaires for measuring human emotions to study anxiety and depression as well as to investigate patients' attitudes about their physicians. Assessment of these kinds of data was made possible because the "Institute developed the first facility in the Medical Center devoted entirely to problems of experimental design and design development. . . . Practical consultation on problems of data analysis has been provided to an ever-expanding group of professional colleagues within the Medical Center . . . ." Work was beginning on mathematical models of behavior using early types of computers. In order to understand the meaning of their research findings, experiments had to be carefully designed and resulting data subject to statistical analysis.

During its opening period, Institute staff had performed teaching duties in the departments of psychiatry, biochemistry, pharmacology, microbiology, medicine, pediatrics, neurology, obstetrics and gynecology, and ophthalmology in the School of Medicine and in the School of Nursing, the School of Dentisrry, and the Indianapolis Division of Indiana University as well as in the Department of Mental Health throughout the state. Nine predoctoral and five postdoctoral fellows completed one or more years of research training and expcrience; seventy-two student research fellows completed a minimum of three months each of supervised research training by institute staff. Staff had provided lectures to physicians' groups around the state and for state facilities. Two hundred and four papers and twenty-one books, monographs, and book chapters had been published.

Research at the institute was leading to understanding the "intangible" elements "which are the province of psychiatry," as Nurnberger said. Continuing studies at the institute would compare animal models and research about patients to elucidate further the causes and treatments of psychiatric disorders. Such studies had been impossible at the time the Pathological Department was built in the 1890s, but now at the Institute of Psychiatric Research in the 1960s, Edenharter's dream was becoming reality.

Notes

1. *Indianapolis Star*, May 12, 1953.

2. *Time*, October 18, 1954.

3. J. N. Hingtgen, "The Institute of Psychiatric Research of the Department of Psychiatry and the Indiana University School of Medicine: The Past Prepares for the Future (1956–2007)." Unpublished.

4. *Indianapolis Star*, December 4, 1956.

5. J. I. Nurnberger, "The Psychiatric Research Institute—A Statement of Aims and Purposes," *Quarterly Bulletin of Indiana University Medical Center* 19 (1957): 21–25.

6. Institute of Psychiatric Research, *First Annual Report of the Institute of Psychiatric Research of the Department of Psychiatry, Indiana University Medical Center and the Division of Mental Health, the State of Indiana, July 1, 1957, to June 30, 1958.*

7. J. I. Nurnberger, C. B. Ferster, and J. P. Brady, *An Introduction to the Science of Human Behavior* (New York: Appleton-Century-Crofts, 1963).

8. Institute of Psychiatric Research, *First Annual Report.*

9. Ibid.

10. Institute of Psychiatric Research, *First Annual Report*; *Third Annual Report of the Institute of Psychiatric Research of the Department of Psychiatry, Indiana University Medical Center and the Division of Mental Health, the State of Indiana, July 1, 1959 to June 30, 1960.*

11. Institute of Psychiatric Research, *Second Annual Report of the Institute of Psychiatric Research of the Department of Psychiatry, Indiana University Medical Center and the Division of Mental Health, the State of Indiana, July 1, 1958 to June 30, 1959.*

12. Ibid.

13. Institute of Psychiatric Research, *Third Annual Report.*

14. J. N. Hingtgen, "The Institute of Psychiatric Research . . . 1956–2007."

15. Ibid.

16. J. N. Hingtgen, personal communication.

17. Institute of Psychiatric Research, *Second Annual Report.*

18. M. H. Aprison and C. B. Ferster, "Serotonin and Behavior," *Recent Advances in Biological Psychiatry* 3 (1961): 151–63.

19. Institute of Psychiatric Research, *Second Annual Report*; Institute of Psychiatric Research, *Third Annual Report.*

20. Ibid.

21. Ibid.

22. Institute of Psychiatric Research, *Fifth Annual Report, July 1, 1961 to June 30, 1962.*

23. Ibid.

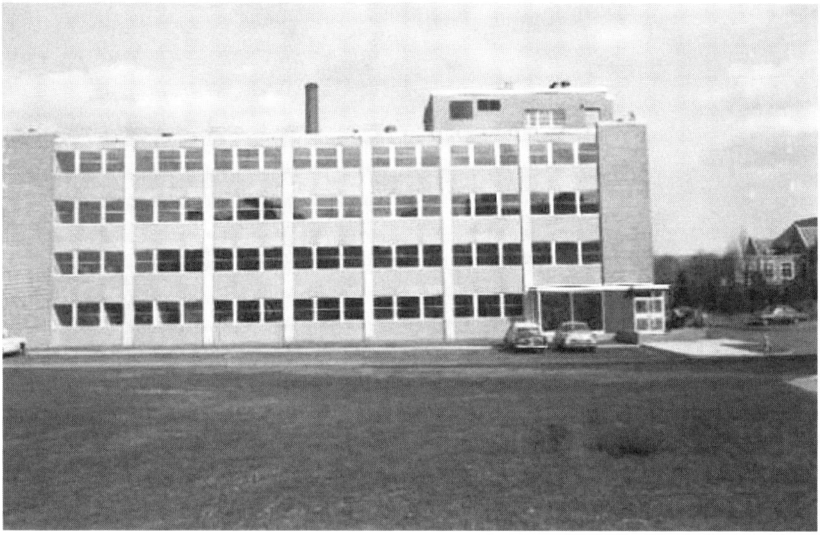

The Institute of Psychiatric Research (IPR) in its early days, the late 1950s. It was designed by architects Daggett, Naegele and Daggett. The firm had also designed its neighbor Larue Carter Hospital a few years earlier.

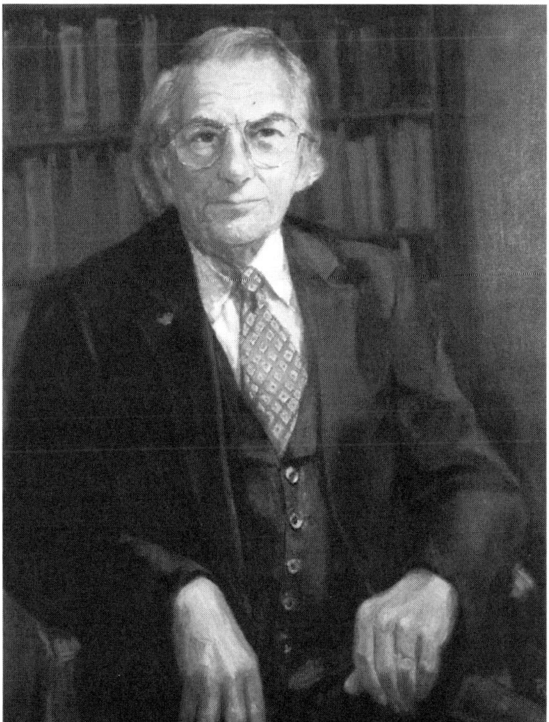

Biochemist Dr. Morris Aprison, pioneer in neurotransmitter research, a gateway for understanding psychiatric disorders and potential treatments. His laboratory was in the IPR. Aprison's publications appeared in prestigious journals from 1952–1996. He continued research and teaching until he was in his late 70s.

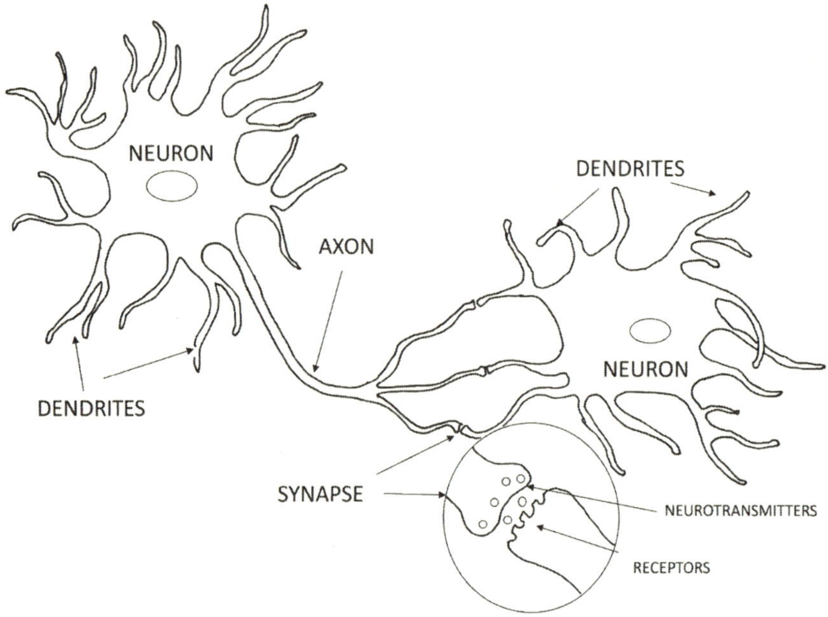

When a nerve cell (neuron) is stimulated by another cell, chemical messengers (neurotransmitters) are released from tiny vesicles at the end of the axon. They pass through the space between cells (synapse) and attach to receptors on the dendrites or cell body of another neuron, stimulating chemical reactions that send an electric current down the axon of that cell. This drawing, which is not to scale, shows a synapse multiplied many thousands of times. *[See pp.61-2.]*

Governor George N. Craig, 1953–1957 ran on a platform that included reform of mental health treatment. This portrait is by Hoosier artist Frances Norris Streit.

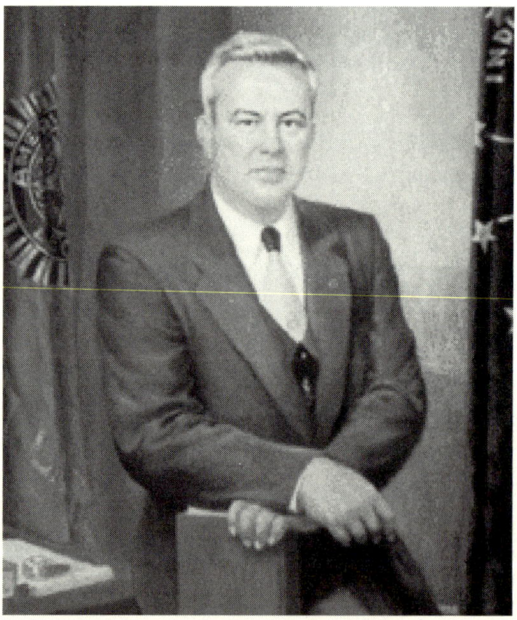

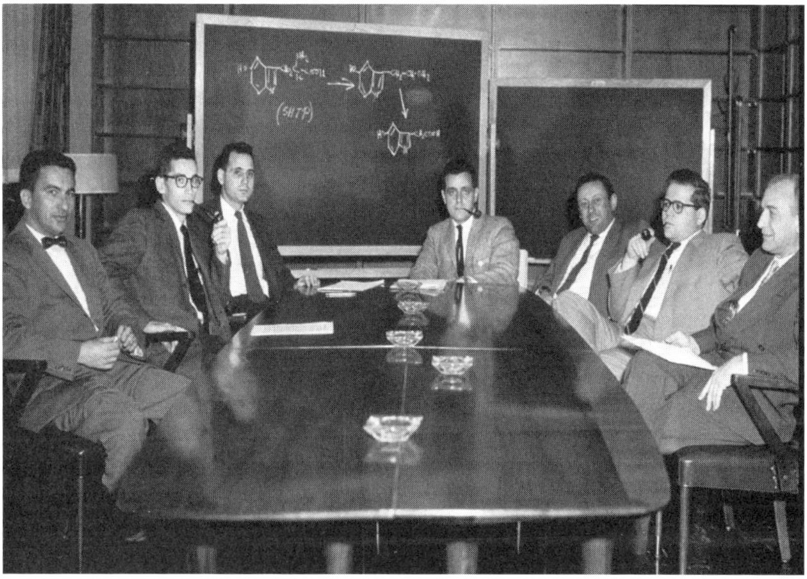

An informal Wednesday morning research conference at IPR (l-r) Drs. Morris Aprison, Richard McCaman, Charles Ferster, Marvin Zucherman, Harold Persky, Harvard L. Armus, and John Nurnberger, Sr.

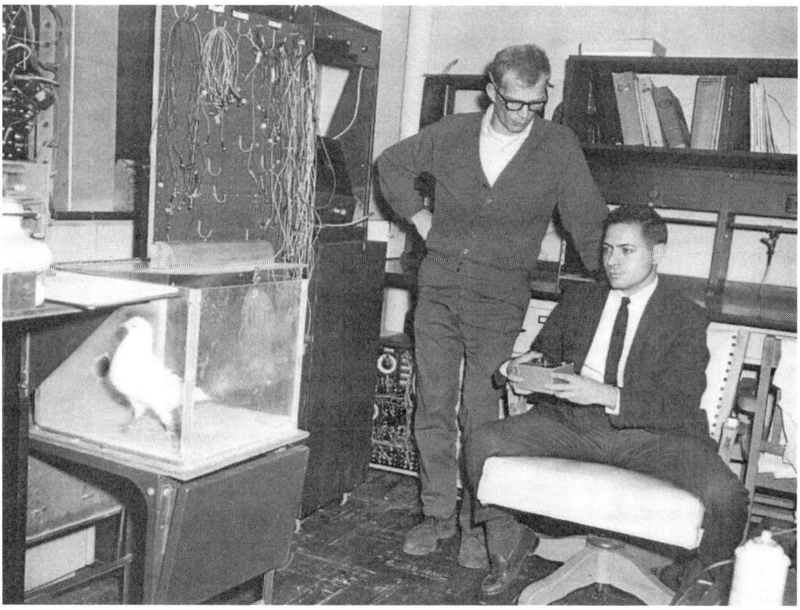

Dr. Charles Ferster (standing) and Joseph Zimmerman, PhD, Research Associate in Experimental Psychology, with a pigeon in the box where it can peck a disc for food. Aprison and Ferster found that the amount of serotonin in the pigeon's brain controlled the frequency of pecking.

5
A Hospital is an Extension of the Community
Larue Carter Hospital II

Donald Moore, MD, mentioned in the previous chapter as cooperating with the institute, was the longest-serving superintendent to date at Larue Carter Hospital, serving from 1955 to 1980. Moore's family, originally from upstate New York, had moved to Michigan in the mid-1800s. They were farmers but had an abiding interest in books and education. Moore grew and matured at a time of great social and economic change, and his fascination with how people responded to these changes led to his choice of a career in medicine and psychiatry. Growing up in Kalamazoo, where his father taught economics at a local college, many of his early memories were of the family farm, his enjoyment of the Boy Scouts, and exploring Michigan's wonderful lakes and forests. Moore attended undergraduate and medical schools at the University of Michigan, where he was awarded the MD degree in 1938. He completed his psychiatric residency at the Ypsilanti State Hospital. Joining the army in World War II, he served primarily in Texas. After his discharge from active duty, he was recruited by the Veterans' Affairs Hospital psychiatry program in Louisville, Kentucky.

Moore was recruited to Indiana University shortly before Nurnberger became chairman of the Department of Psychiatry. At IU School of Medicine Moore rose through the academic ranks quickly and was appointed professor of psychiatry in the late 1960s. He and his family—wife Carolla, whose newspaper work prior to their marriage allowed her to edit Moore's writings, and four children—occupied an apartment on the fourth floor of the original Tenth Street Carter Hospital throughout his tenure as superintendent, just as superintendents like Edenharter and Bahr, at Central State Hospital, had lived on the grounds there.

Moore co-authored scientific papers addressing most of the major clinical psychiatric issues of his day. He was chair of the editorial board for the American Psychiatric Association journal, *Hospital and Community Psychiatry*, in the 1960s. He was also active on the American Board of Psychiatry and Neurology and headed an examining team for the oral board examination for many years. Highly involved in administrative psychiatry, he wrote several articles on this topic and was a founding member of the Association of Medical Superintendents of Mental Hospitals (now the American Association of Psychiatric Administrators), serving as its president in 1966–1967.[1]

As an administrator Moore was fond of saying, "Don't pass anxiety downwards." In line with that philosophy, he sheltered the Carter Hospital medical staff and others from the many political storms that raged during his tenure.[2] He fully supported the developing research program at Carter Hospital despite strong opposition from traditionally oriented staff—those who preferred a psychoanalytic approach rather than new medications and those who worried about research involving patients, even if it promised results that would be to their ultimate benefit. There was a conviction among some staff that new faculty who were doing research on medications and convulsive therapies as treatments should not be allowed to use psychotherapy as a treatment.

Moore enjoyed the challenge of creating new positions and programs previously unknown in the state, overcoming resistance at all levels of authority and making resources available whenever he could. His particular talent lay in his ability to persuade state officials to fund mental health, not only for Carter Hospital, but also for the other state hospitals. Like Edenharter, Bahr, and Larue Carter before him, he kept in touch with politicians and emphasized the importance of any new programs he proposed. He was a passionate supporter of the psychiatry residency program, obtaining hard money funding at a time when this was a rarity. These funding streams continue to support psychiatric residency education at Indiana University to this day. He also worked tirelessly to obtain JCAHO (Joint Commission on Accreditation of Health Care Organizations) accreditation for Carter Hospital, holding the hospital to high clinical standards and increasing eligibility for federal funding.

Aware of the importance of developing positive relationships with important public informational sources, he cultivated the major media of the time: the *Indianapolis Star* and the *Indianapolis News.* He was described in a newspaper article as possessing "a hearty optimism. His cheerful good humor hardly seemed to go with the complex job of administering the key institution in Indiana's mental health program." Moore expressed his view, "A hospital is an extension of the community, and not a separate one. We foster this philosophy by taking almost any group for a tour of the hospital." Retaining archaic stereotypes and memories from B movies, visitors often expected to see patients in restraints and in locked cells, but Moore showed them "the ward where the disturbed patients live. All of the rooms are similar [to those for other patients]." Rarely were patients placed alone in seclusion rooms. There were no straightjackets, and restraints were rarely used.[3]

While Moore was addressing stigma against psychiatric patients on a local level, a national event began the long journey toward erasing the stereotype of psychiatric illness for the country as a whole. In 1972 Senator George McGovern, running against President Richard Nixon in the presidential election, suggested Senator Thomas Eagleton as his running mate. The media publicized the fact that Eagleton had been hospitalized for major depression and had had electroconvulsive ("shock") treatments. Eagleton was replaced on the ticket, but for the first time there was a great deal of publicity about the diagnosis of depression and use of "shock" treatments. Prominent psychiatrists were quoted with positive opinions about the prognosis of the illness and the value and safety of the treatments. Meanwhile, Moore in Indianapolis had been demonstrating to the public that state psychiatric hospitals did not have to be places of mystery and horror. Inroads were being made into public attitudes about psychiatric disorders and treatment.

At the time, 88 percent of patients at Carter Hospital signed in voluntarily (avoiding a commitment hearing before a probate judge), which Moore credited to the diminishing stigma of psychiatric disorders. He had recently reviewed outcomes of one thousand patients who had been discharged. Nine hundred twenty-five had resumed normal lives at home. Seventy were in treatment elsewhere in the state, some of whom would eventually return home. Five had died, Moore reported. "We're not satisfied with only 92.5 per cent going home. We would like to get the other 7.5 per cent home, too, so we can put ourselves out of business some day." He noted that most of the 7.5 percent had schizophrenia, a disorder that is still difficult to treat in the twenty-first century. [4]

Individuals with schizophrenia suffer from disorders of thinking and perception of the world around them. They often see and hear things that are not there (hallucinations) and are convinced that certain strange ideas are true in spite of all evidence to the contrary (delusions). Hallucinations and delusions are often of a disturbing or even frightening nature: someone is trying to harm them, bizarre alterations are taking place in their bodies, secret messages are being sent to them via television, and the like. Trivial occurrences are interpreted as proof of their fears, e.g., someone turning on an outside light is interpreted as a signal to foreign spies. Social skills and occupational functioning are seriously compromised. Because manifestations of the illness first appear in adolescence, educational progress might be cut short. Verbalizations often don't make sense, such as "I feel that everything is sort of related to everybody and that some people are far more susceptible to this theory of relativity than others because of either having previous ancestors connected in some way or other with places or things, or because of believing, or by leaving a trail behind when you walk through a room you know."[5]

Behavior might be so bizarre that no one would doubt that

the individual is severely disturbed. Although symptoms might wax and wane, the illness tends to be chronic. The many antipsychotic medications developed over the years since the 1950s and the psychosocial therapies aimed at improving functioning in real-life situations are quite helpful—individuals with schizophrenia no longer vegetate for years on back wards of state psychiatric hospitals—but no complete cure is available as yet.

One of the outstanding collaborations between Larue Carter Hospital and its neighbor, the Institute of Psychiatric Research, was the collaboration of behavioral psychologist Ferster with Marian DeMyer, MD, at the hospital's residential treatment unit for disturbed children, one of the few centers in the country for studying what was then called "childhood schizophrenia," now known as autism. In 1961 DeMyer and Nurnberger received an $800,000 federal grant to continue the studies.[6] DeMyer was a pioneer in research about autism, having identified it as a neurological/developmental disorder rather than a psychological problem caused by inadequate parents as some had proposed. She received an award from the director of the National Institute of Mental Health in 1974. Her 1979 book summarizes decades of her work.[7]

Ferster constructed a controlled environment in which simple activity could be sustained with autistic children on DeMyer's children's residential treatment unit at Larue Carter Hospital. They were able to extend the behavioral repertoire of these children and were beginning to work with ways to improve perception, an area of major deficit in autism. Within a year they were able to help severely autistic children maintain ordered behavior for periods of time.[8] In 1962 Ferster took a leave of absence to develop a laboratory in College Park, Maryland. Joseph Hingtgen, who had received his PhD in psychology from Loyola University in Chicago, joined the institute staff. Hingtgen continued the research with DeMyer at Larue Carter Hospital.

Hingtgen described work with autistic children:

> A major deficiency . . . of autistic children is their lack of social interaction with their peers. A method was developed for shaping cooperative responses in autistic children by using reinforcement techniques in a controlled setting. Six low-functioning autistic children, who had been observed to initiate little or no social interaction with their peers, were trained [in pairs] to operate a lever to obtain coins which could be used to obtain candy, crackers and cereal from vending machines . . . cooperative responses were shaped in succeeding sessions so that eventually children learned to alternate (take turns) in order to operate the coin lever. The results indicated that it was possible to shape cooperative responses in the pairs within an average of 23 sessions. Physical contacts and vocal responses between partners, although not directly reinforced, were seen to increase beyond what had been observed on the ward. A subsequent study which more directly reinforced vocal responses and appropriate physical contact in nonverbal, low functioning autistic children during 46 daily sessions, was able to show a significant increase in these responses outside the experimental sessions.[9]

These results suggested techniques that could be used for increasing social and vocal behavior in low-functioning autistic children. Another deficit in these children is lack of imitative behavior:

> The establishment of imitative responses . . . [might] significantly increase the overall range of behaviors . . . [and] would suggest that even for low functioning autistic children, some of the deficits associated with autism may not be irreversible . . . two mute, low-functioning autistic children, who had not shown any improvement following various types of traditionally oriented therapy, were individually given 6 hours of daily training sessions for 21 days. . . . During sessions food treats, water and release from physical restraint were used to reinforce three types of imitative behaviors, progressing from simple to more complex skills: (1) general use of body including head, fingers, arms; (2) use of

> objects such as buttons, scissors, toys; and (3) vocalizations. . . . Five months following the initial training period the children had progressed beyond imitative responding, and were doing such things as printing letters of the alphabet using a visual or auditory cue, cutting out figures with scissors, and naming various pictures and objects . . . a short-term intensive imitative training period might be effective in establishing a large number of behaviors which can be used by parents, teachers and others. . . .

In establishing new behaviors in some low-functioning autistic children, it sometimes appears that the child simply will not try. The child becomes angry, silly, ritualistic, affectionate, or does not respond. The low-level incapacity of these children, likely associated with neurobiological deficits, contributes to the apparent negativism. This difficulty learning new behaviors can be changed by a persistent approach that not only rewards attention and responding, but which makes the consequences of nonresponding (e.g., withholding food treats) more unpleasant than those of responding. Periods of "won't try" are replaced by a "will try" attitude, and the child becomes focused on the task at hand. It is important not only to raise motivation, but also to give training in the most basic skills. These early pioneering studies under the leadership of Marian DeMyer led to the development of more treatment programming for autistic children and improved the therapeutic outlook considerably for greater numbers of these children. They continued this pattern of very carefully designed research on improving social behavior.

A 1981 review, dedicated to the memory of Ferster, who had recently died as well as to the famous child psychiatrist Leo Kanner, who had first identified the syndrome of autism, included confirmation of DeMyers's research that autism is a neurodevelopmental disorder best treated by a behavioral/educational approach and that parents of autistic children had "no psychopathology which conceivably could induce the disorder."[10] It was a tremendous relief to an entire community of tortured parents and set the stage for positive rehabilitative strategies.

In 1966 Nurnberger hired Joyce Small, MD, as research director and Iver Small, MD, as medical director, a husband-and-wife team originally from Canada, working at the time at Washington University in St. Louis. They would develop the psychopharmacological research program at Larue Carter Hospital to study the many new treatments becoming available for psychiatric illnesses. In the years to come, in over 120 papers describing rigorously conceived research about convulsive treatments and psychotropic medications, they provided valuable evidence about all aspects of these modalities. Joyce Small received the National Institute of Mental Health Merit Program Award in 1990. The Smalls also provided teaching for medical students and residents and consultation for clinicians interested in the latest data about newer medication.

Joyce Small specialized in electroencephalography, the study of electrical activity in the various areas of the brain via electrodes placed on the scalp and attached to a recording device. Electroencephalogram (EEG) recordings of "brain waves" (oscillations) show four patterns of oscillations called alpha, beta, gamma, and theta. These are stable and are largely determined genetically. One of the concerns in the 1970s and 1980s was refining psychiatric diagnoses so that research could be done more carefully on specific illnesses and treatments (e.g., that antidepressants could be used for patients with carefully diagnosed major depressive disorder, not just with anyone who felt sad) and so that the new medications could be more readily tailored to individual patients. In one study of 759 patients originally diagnosed with schizophrenia at Larue Carter Hospital, newer diagnostic criteria, admitting EEGs, and outcomes were compared. One-third of patients were no longer diagnosed with the usually chronic illness of schizophrenia. Their diagnoses now included affective (mood) disorders and disorders due to medical illnesses (e.g., delirium, dementia), many of which would be expected to have a better prognosis than schizophrenia. EEGs predicted prognosis, or outcome. For example, mean alpha frequencies were slower in patients with schizophrenia. Follow-up diagnoses ten or more years after admission were significantly correlated with admission EEGs.[11] EEG studies had previously been used primarily to study illnesses related to neurological conditions or schizophrenia. The Smalls were applying this technique in new and creative ways, in this case exploring possibilities of using EEGs as predictors of illness rather than just studying individual illnesses. In 2003 Joyce Small received a Career Award from the EEG and Clinical Neuroscience Society for leadership in psychiatry and her exceptional contribution to EEG research and its clinical applications.

Research Design—Controls

One of the problems with any study of new treatments is that many illnesses in all specialties of medicine—even if severe—get well without specific treatment. If a patient recovers after a specific treatment, was recovery the result of treatment, or would it have occurred with no treatment? For this reason, studies of new treatments often use "controls." For example, half the patients in a study (the control group) are given a placebo or harmless pill with no therapeutic effect, and the other half of patients are given the new medicine. Both placebo and new medicine are prepared in similar capsules or tablets. The research is "double-blind"—neither patients nor staff know which bottles have placebo and which contain the new medicine. Only the research scientists have the code of which bottles contain what. Patients' symptoms are rated with standardized questionnaires by staff who do not know who are controls and who are getting the new medicine. At the end of the study, patient improvement (fewer or no symptoms) is noted, and the code is broken to see whether or not those patients who improved were much more likely to have received the new medicine. Statistical evaluation of the data establishes whether or not the new medicine is better than placebo. Once there are medicines known to improve a given disorder, one of them would be used instead of placebo to see whether or not a new medicine is better than an established treatment.

Nowhere is careful research about new treatments

more important than in treatment of mood disorders (major depressive disorder, bipolar disorder). Episodes of the disorders might remit in days, weeks, months, or years. Therefore it is very important to design carefully any research about treatment effectiveness.

Many variations of convulsive therapies—still the most effective therapy for mood disorders when medications and psychotherapy fail—were being tried. The Smalls' group at Carter Hospital studied these newer methods to determine whether or not they improved on traditional treatment. Electrodes for electroconvulsive treatment (ECT, electroshock, EST) had traditionally been placed bilaterally on the patient's temples. Now some suggested that unilateral placement on the non-dominant side would be just as effective and might not cause as much temporary recent memory loss.[12] The experiment was double-blinded by placing electrode paste on both temples of those receiving unilateral placement of electrodes. When patients returned to the ward, staff would not know who had received which treatment. The unilateral modification was found generally not to be as effective as bilateral electrode placement.

Another innovation was producing seizures with flurothyl (Indoklon), an ether that produces convulsions. This study's controls had to be carefully devised. For example, when comparing flurothyl and ECT, the researchers put a few drops of the ether on the hospital gowns of those receiving ECT so that the odor would be present and placed electrodes on the temples of those receiving fluorothyl so that the electrode paste would be present. Thus patients and ward staff were blind to who had received which treatment and evaluations of improvement would be blind as to treatment modality.[13]

Traditional ECT proved superior to the newer modifications. Such studies were invaluable to clinicians throughout the country who might, it was hoped, consider changing to new treatments that might not, in fact, be as valuable as initially thought. Currently even newer techniques of brain stimulation are being used for treatment in the Department of Psychiatry, such as repetitive transcranial magnetic stimulation (rTMS).

The Carter Hospital group also spearheaded research to elucidate the mechanisms of action of electroconvulsive therapy (ECT). The number of possible mechanisms was considerably decreased as studies narrowed the range of likely mechanisms. Neuropsychological testing indicated right (brain) hemisphere dysfunctions in affective illness that resolved more in patients for whom ECT proved beneficial than in those whose depressions did not improve much with ECT. Transient left-sided EEG slowing was associated with positive ECT response. The authors concluded that their data supported the hypothesis that in patients with mood disorders, ECT restores equilibrium between activity in the two halves of the brain with enhancement of right brain function and dampening of the left.[14]

They studied the effects of ECT on the heart in patients with no cardiac conditions and concluded "[s]timulation produced by ECT did not induce arrhythmias in these patients without heart disease."[15] They used the pituitary hormone ACTH versus placebo to study whether, as postulated, it would diminish recent memory loss with ECT and found that it did not.[16] During the decades of their research, many aspects of convulsive therapy were studied, providing a major contribution to the treatment literature both as to what methods were most effective and as to possible side effects.

New medications for treatment of severe psychiatric disorders became available during the 1950s and 1960s. Many of these administered to a variety of patients were studied by the research group at Carter Hospital, fulfilling the original goal of providing the best and most up-to-date treatments for patients there as well as those elsewhere when psychiatrists read psychiatric journals in which Carter studies were published. Larue Carter Hospital often admitted patients who had not improved with standard treatment. Studies were carried out to determine how best to benefit these patients, often with the latest medications available. For example, the anticonvulsants carbamazepine, divalproate, and clonazepam were studied in comparison to lithium carbonate and ECT, existing treatments for mania at the time.[17] Anticonvulsants are now an important part of the treatment armamentarium for mania: like lithium they provide remission of symptoms in many patients and improvement in others.

Some of the newer medications were being used in combinations. In a collaborative study with other institutions focused on prevention of recurrent episodes of mood disorders, patients with either major depression or bipolar disorder (depressions and manias) were given the antidepressant imipramine or the mood stabilizer lithium carbonate or a combination of the two. In patients with bipolar disorder, lithium carbonate prevented both manic and depressive episodes. Imipramine prevented recurrence in patients with major depression. The combination of drugs did not improve on the single drug. Only lithium prevented manic episodes.[18] Many of the carefully researched findings of the Carter Hospital group became common practice for psychiatric treatment around the country.

In spite of modern settings for patient treatment, support for nationally recognized research, and education of young doctors for Indiana, Moore became a target for complaints to the governor. Moore theorized that living onsite at the hospital and having to be available at all hours of the day and night for hospital issues secured him many hours of "compensatory time" to return to his beloved Michigan. He owned a cottage there and could be available by phone, as well as always appointing an "acting superintendent" to act on his behalf when he was not in Indianapolis. Someone, however, began calling the Statehouse on a regular basis whenever Moore was away, asking what the governor was going to do about Moore's "lengthy paid vacations." The governor delegated the problem to his commissioner of mental health, Dr. William Murray.

Murray had experienced some sort of problem at Newcastle State Hospital early in his career there, and Moore had stepped in to help. They found they shared many things in common and had become friends, and so Moore hoped Commissioner Murray might be able to defend him against the governor's office. That proved wrong, and Moore was fired, to be followed soon by Murray's departure. Some wondered if they had had each other fired.

Both men continued to be active in the psychiatric community. Murray was very proud of the fact that, while he was mental health commissioner, he had overseen the development of Indiana's community mental health system. This was a federal mandate begun during the Kennedy presidency. Community mental health centers were supposed to enable states to move the care of those with psychiatric disorders who could not afford private treatment out of their large state hospitals and entirely into the community. Indiana decided on a system of thirty-one mental health centers (one of which was never completed), scattered strategically around the state, and Murray had seen the system nearly completed before leaving office. He didn't go to work in one of his centers, though, instead entering private practice in Indianapolis. Upon his death, his extensive library, including many books important to the history of psychiatry's development in his time, was donated to Carter Hospital and is now housed in the "Murray Room" at the hospital. Moore remained active in organized psychiatry both locally and nationally for nearly twenty additional years, dying in Indianapolis in 1999 at age eight-five. His portrait, along with those of several other former Carter superintendents, including Moore, now hangs in the board room at Carter Hospital, uniting the two men posthumously and recognizing, in a way, the friendship they shared earlier in their careers and the zeal both carried throughout life for improving the care of the mentally ill.

Notes

1. J. G. Small and I. F. Small, unpublished biographical notes.
2. John Gerhart, "Behind the Medics: Larue Carter Chief Runs Calm Hospital—Mental Illness Stigma Easing," *Indianapolis Times*, October 24, 1960.
3. Ibid.
4. Ibid.

5. E. Slater and M. Roth, *Mayer-Gross Slater and Roth Clinical Psychiatry* (London: Bailliere, Tindall, and Cassell, 1969), 267.
6. Clipping file, Larue Carter Hospital library.
7. M. K. DeMyer, *Parents and Children in Autism* (Washington, DC: V. H. Winston and Sons, 1979).
8. Institute of Psychiatric Research, *Second Annual Report of the Institute of Psychiatric Research of the Department of Psychiatry, Indiana University Medical Center and the Division of Mental Health, the State of Indiana, July 1, 1958 to June 30, 1959*; Institute of Psychiatric Research, *Third Annual Report of the Institute of Psychiatric Research of the Department of Psychiatry, Indiana University Medical Center and the Division of Mental Health, the State of Indiana, July 1, 1959 to June 30, 1960.*
9. J. N. Hingtgen, personal communication summarizing the following publications: J. N. Hingtgen, B. J. Sanders, and M. K. DeMyer, "Shaping Cooperative Responses in Early Childhood Schizophrenics," in *Case Studies in Behavior Modification*, ed. L. Ullmann and L. Krasner (New York: Holt, Rinehart, and Winston, 1965), 130–38; J. N. Hingtgen and F. C. Trost, "Shaping Cooperative Responses in Early Childhood Schizophrenics: II Reinforcement of Mutual Physical Contact and Vocal Responses," in *Control of Human Behavior*, ed. R. Ulrich, T. Stachnik, and J. Mabry (Chicago: Scott, Foresman, and Co., 1966), 110–13; J. N. Hingtgen, S. K. Coulter, and D. W. Churchill, "Intensive Reinforcement of Imitative Behavior in Mute Autistic Children," *Archives of General Psychiatry* 17 (1967): 36–43; J. N. Hingten and S. K. Coulter, "Auditory Control of Operant Behavior in Mute Autistic Children," *Perceptual and Motor Skills* 25 (1967): 561–65; J. N. Hingtgen and D. W. Churchill, "Identification of Perceptual Limitations in Mute Autistic Children," *Archives of General Psychiatry* 21 (1969): 68–71.
10. M. K. DeMyer, J. N. Hingtgen, and R. K. Jackson, "Infantile Autism Reviewed: A Decade of Research," *Schizophrenia Bulletin* 7 (1981): 388–451.
11. J. G. Small, V. Milstein, P. H. Sharpley, M. Klapper, and I. F. Small, "Electroencephalographic Findings in Relation to Diagnostic Constructs in Psychiatry," *Biological Psychiatry* 19 (1984): 471–87.
12. J. G. Small, I. F. Small, and G. E. Gans, "Sensory Evoked Responses with Unilateral Electroconvulsive Treatment," *Electroencephalography and Clinical Neurophysiology* 30 (1971): 164; V. Milstein, J. G. Small, M. H. Klapper, I. F. Small, M. J. Miller, and J. J. Kellams, "Universus Bilateral ECT in the Treatment of Mania," *Convulsive Therapy* 3 (1987): 1–9.
13. J. G. Small, I. F. Small, P. Sharpley, and D. F. Moore, "A Double-Blind Comparative Evaluation of Florothyl and ECT," *Archives of General Phychiatry 19* (1968): 79-86; J.G. Small and I.F. Small, *"Clinical Results: Indoklon versus ECT," Seminars in Psychiatry 4*(1972): 13-26
14. J. G. Small, V. Milstein, M. J. Miller, P. H. Sharpley, I. F. Small, F. W. Malloy, and M. H. Klapper, "Clinical, Neuropsychological, and EEG Evidence

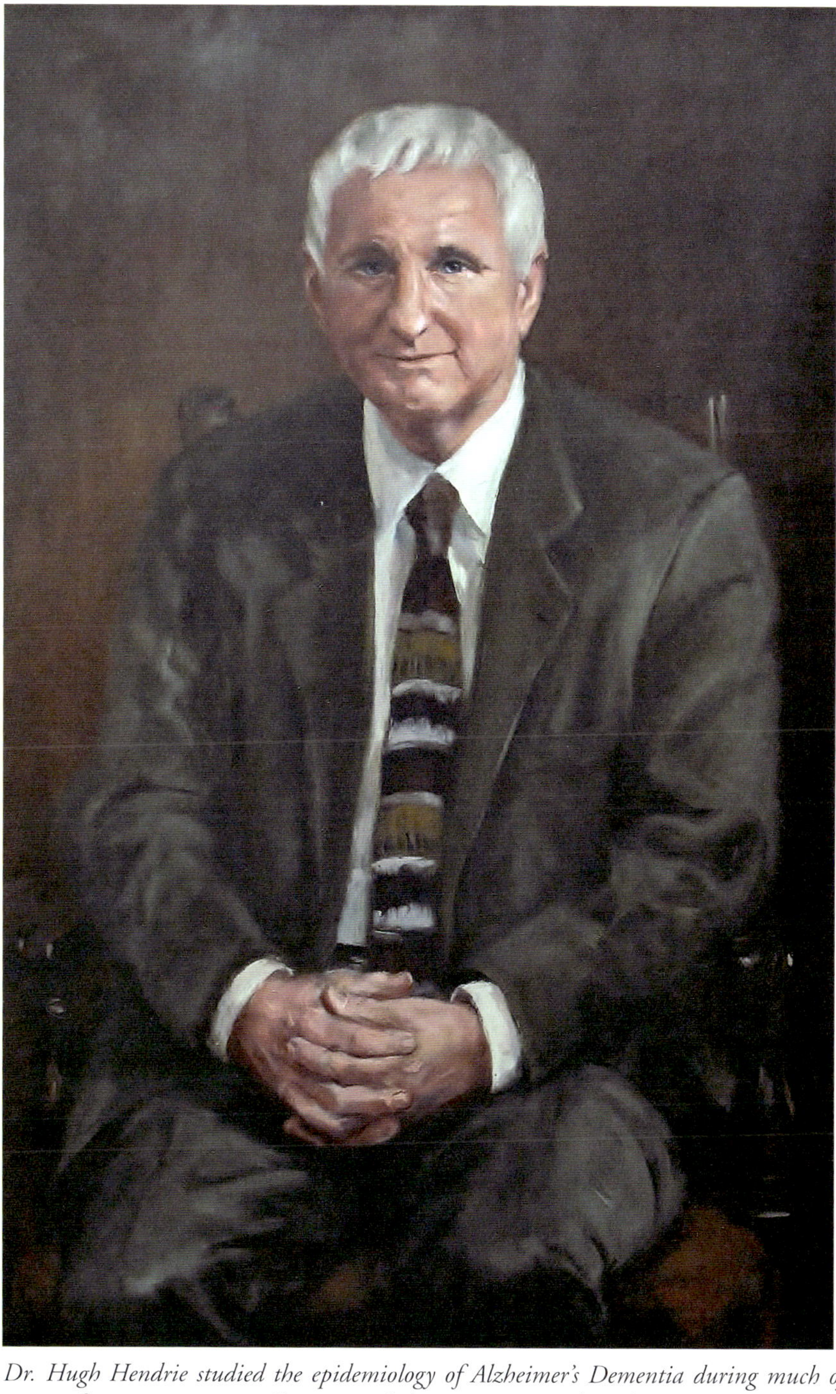

Dr. Hugh Hendrie studied the epidemiology of Alzheimer's Dementia during much of his twenty-five year tenure as Chairman of the Department of Psychiatry, Indiana University School of Medicine, and continued his research after retirement from that position.

Dr. Donald Moore was the second and longest serving superintendent of Larue Carter Hospital. He was the last superintendent at the original hospital to follow the tradition of living on the hospital grounds with his family.

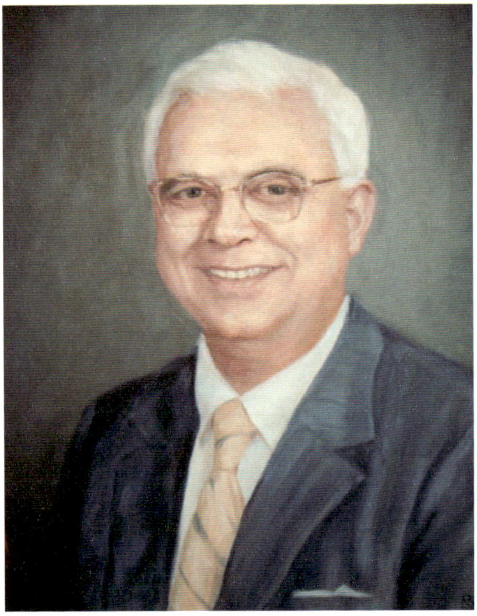

Dr. Juul Nielsen, first superintendent of Larue Carter Memorial Hospital.

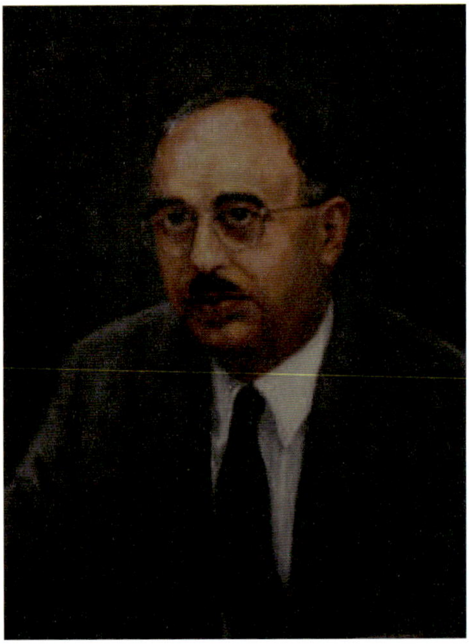

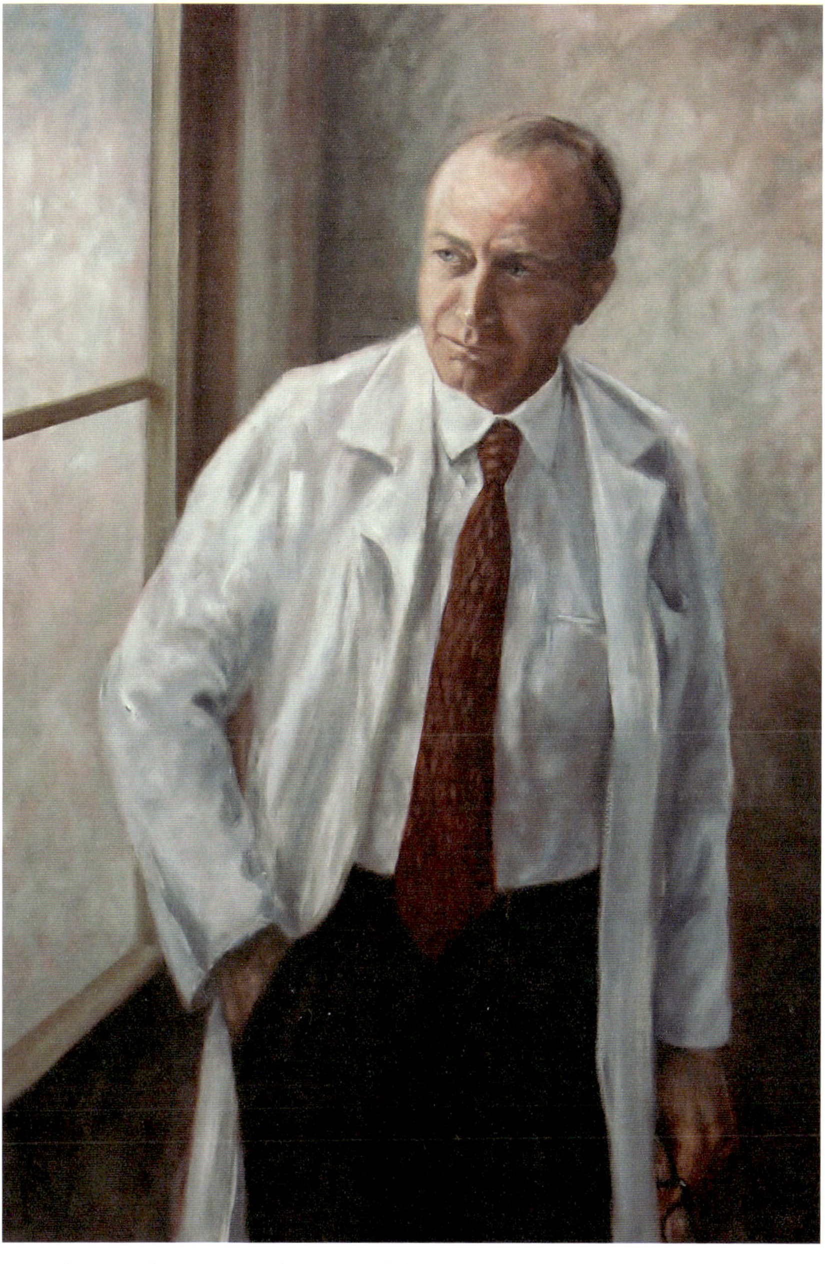

Dr. John Nurnberger, Sr., Chairman of the Department of Psychiatry, Indiana University School of Medicine, and Director of the Institute of Psychiatric Research from 1956 to 1974, exemplified the use of science to improve psychiatric treatment. He was not only a pioneer in neurobiological research in psychiatry in the United States. but also saw the importance of using both medication and psychotherapy in treatment. Both aspects are common today.

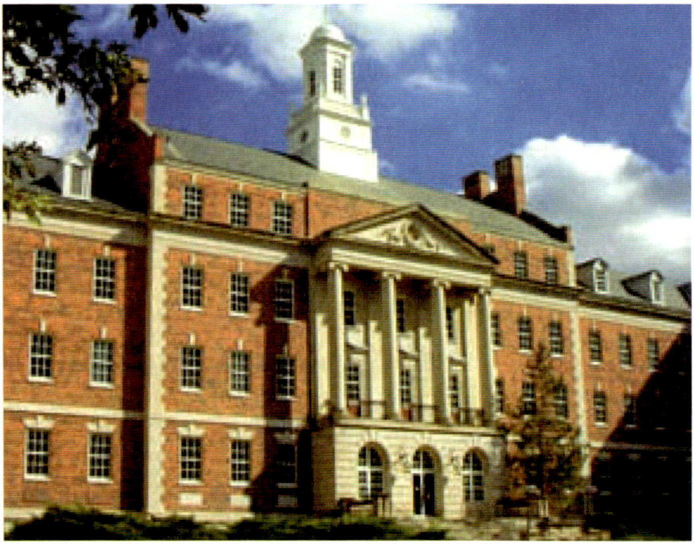

Larue Carter Hospital on Cold Spring Road.

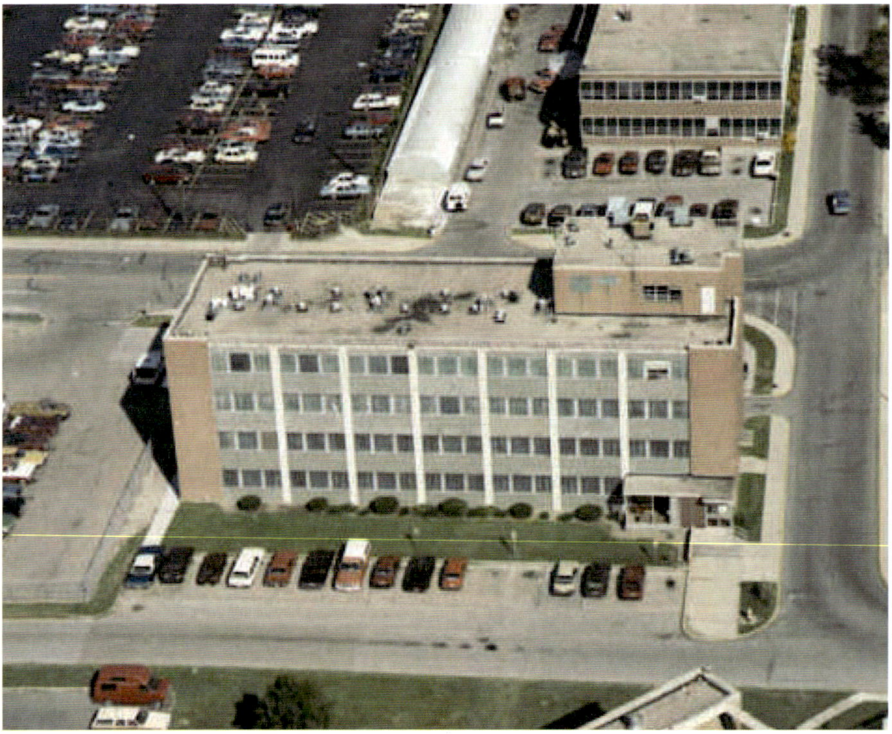

Institute of Psychiatric Research at Indiana University Medical Center, Indianapolis, Indiana.

for Mechanisms of Action of ECT," *Seminars in Psychiatry 4 (1972): 13-26*: 280–91.
15. P. J. Troup, J. G. Small, V. Milstein, I. F. Small, and D. P. Zipes, "Effect of Electroconvulsive Therapy on Cardiac Rhythm, Conduction and Repolarization," *Pacing and Clinical Electrophysiology* 1 (1978): 172–77.
16. J. G. Small, I. F. Small, V. Milstein, and D. A. Dian, "Effects of ACTH 4-10 on ECT-induced Memory Dysfunctions," *Acta Psychiatrica Scandinavia* 55 (1977): 241–50.
17. J. G. Small, "Anticonvulsants in Affective Disorders," *Psychopharmacology Bulletin* 26 (1990): 25–36.
18. R. F. Prien, D. J. Kupfer, P. A. Mansky, J. G. Small, V. B. Tuason, and W. E. Johnson, "Drug Therapy in the Prevention of Recurrences in Unipolar and Bipolar Affective Disorders: Report of the NIMH Collaborative Study Group Comparing Lithium Carbonate, Imipramine, and a Lithium Carbonate-Imipramine Combination," *Archives of General Psychiatry* 41 (1984): 1096–1104.

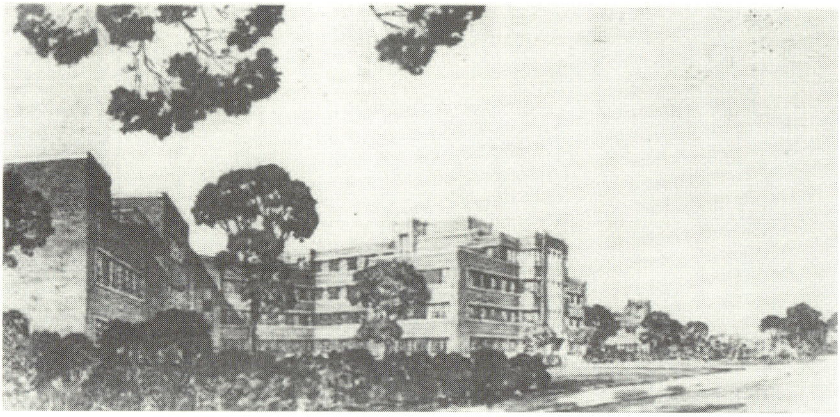

Larue Carter Hospital's original drawing plan. It's interesting to note the optimistically bucolic setting: trees and grassy grounds.

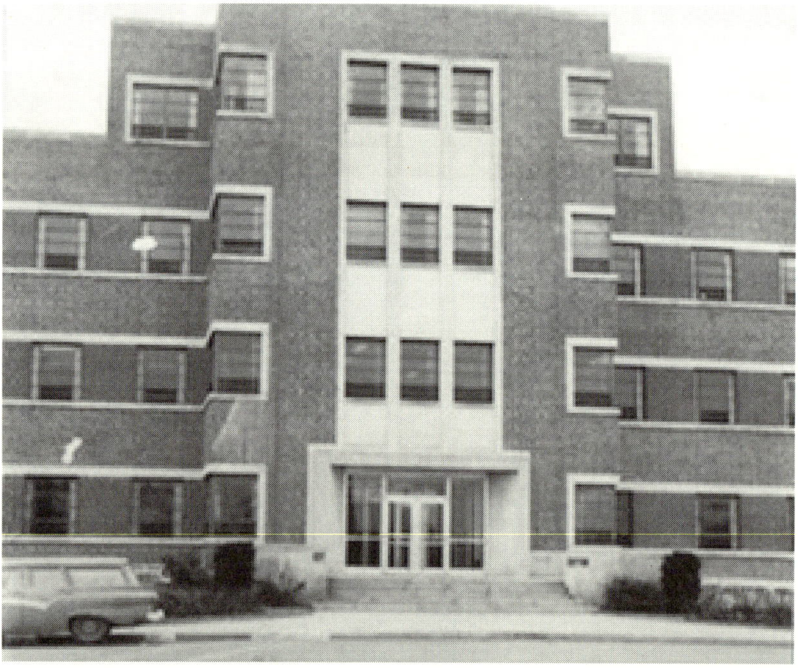

Larue Carter as it was from 1970s to 1980s. Cement and a parking lot.

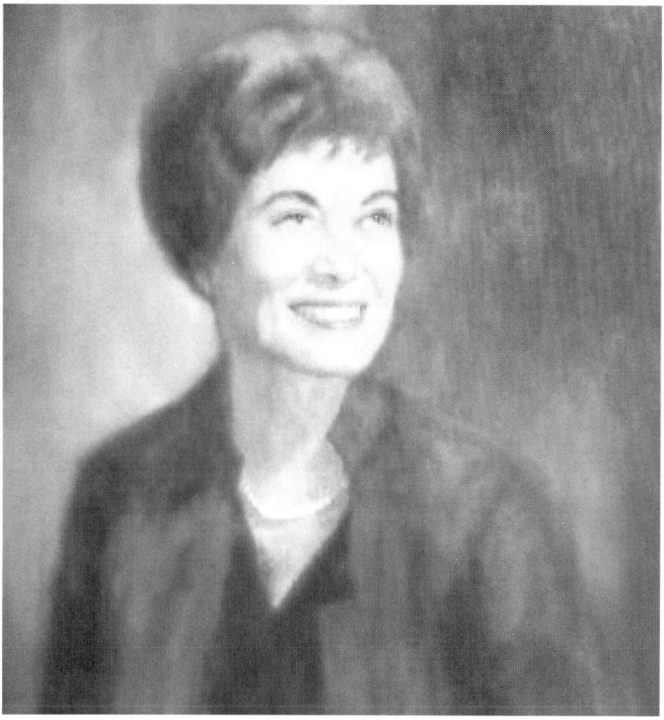

Dr. Marion DeMyer demonstrated that parents were not the cause of autistic disorder in their children and studied behavioral and educational methods to treat autism.

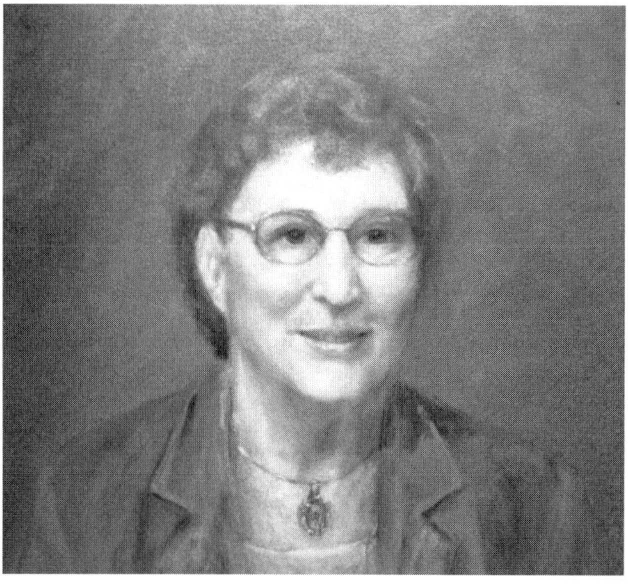

Dr. Joyce Small carefully designed and carried out timely research on the new treatments in psychiatry that were developed in the last half of the twentieth century in order to define how best to use them to treat psychiatric disorders.

Dr. Charles Ferster, a behavioral psychologist, contributed greatly to Aprison's studies of neurotransmitters and DeMyer's work with autistic children.

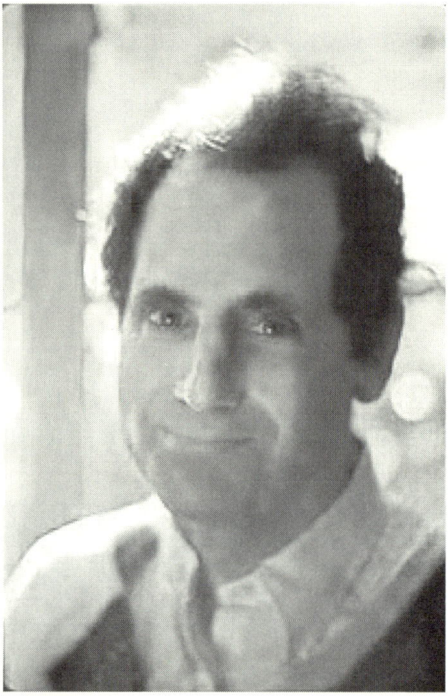

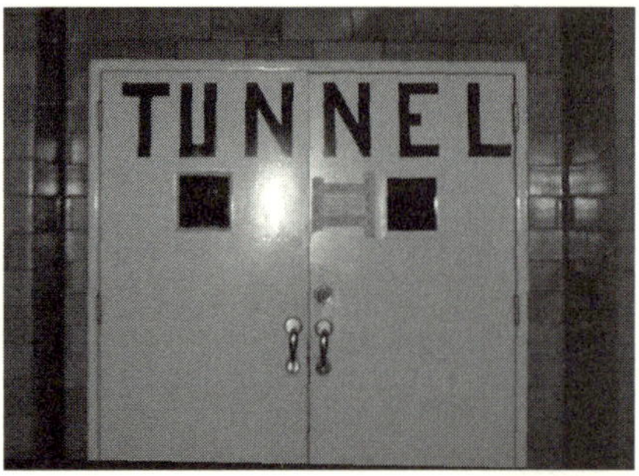

A tunnel connected Larue Carter Hospital with the Institute of Psychiatric Research, part of a system of underground walkways connecting the buildings of Indiana University School of Medicine.

This door led to the ECT Unit E-1, where Carter Hospital psychiatrists administered ECT for many years and studied the results.

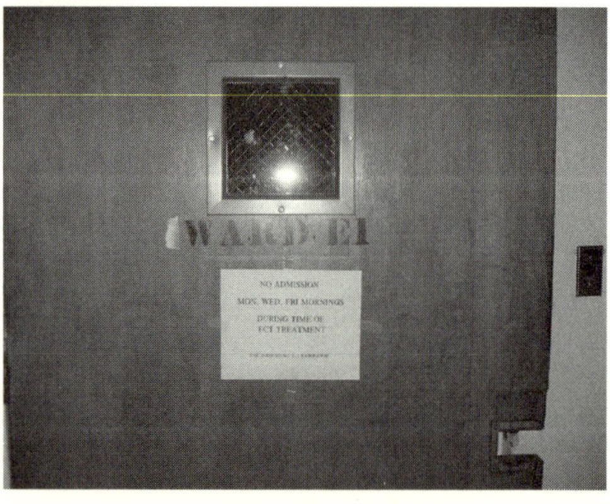

6
Ever More Questions to be Answered

Institute of Psychiatric Research II

Research at the institute continued well beyond the first five years, to the present day. In the 1970s, 80s and 90s, Morris Aprison, using biochemical methods developed in his and other laboratories to measure levels of serotonin and other chemicals in the brain, and Joseph Hingtgen, managing operant conditioning in laboratory animals, studied three neurotransmitters in various areas of the brain under the same experimental conditions as in the previous 5-HTP iproniazid experiments. In these new experiments, only the neurotransmitter serotonin—not the neurotransmitters norepinephrine and dopamine—increased, and the increase was associated with disrupted behavior. Similar studies in rats pressing a lever for a food reward produced the same results. Thus, the research strategy developed to study neurochemical correlates of behavior led to accumulation of evidence to support the landmark finding that ". . . compounds called neurotransmitters . . . have major effects on the behavior of living organisms by their . . . actions on the central nervous system."[1] Researchers had demonstrated a link between neurotransmitters and behavior. Aprison, Hingtgen, and coworkers researched a number of antidepressant medications and observed their effects on their animal model of depression.[2] Administering serotonergic agents directly into a cerebral ventricle (cerebrospinal fluid compartment inside the brain), they demonstrated that the effects of serotonin they had observed were indeed occurring in brain itself and not elsewhere in the body.[3]

Animal models of psychiatric disorders would become a major focus of research at the Institute of Psychiatric Research. These are carefully designed and tested in a variety of ways to determine whether or not they are similar to the human disorder being modeled. Research can be carried out on laboratory animals that would be impossible in human patients, and valuable information obtained that is of benefit to human patients. Obviously, rats are not humans, and there is always the possibility that the model does not fit the particular human disorder in every respect.

At the time of Aprison and Hingtgen's ongoing research, it had been postulated on the basis of studies in patients with major depression that depression resulted from low levels of serotonin in the brain. This did not fit the finding of decreased pecking or lever pressing behavior ("depression") in laboratory animals with elevated serotonin after 5-HTP or iproniazid. To explain the discrepancy in their findings as compared with the work of others, Aprison and Hingtgen suggested that some types of depression might be related to an excess, rather than a deficiency, of serotonin in the brain.[4] Theirs was one of the early animal models of depression and demonstrates some of the difficulties of translating laboratory animal data to clinical situations in patients.

At this point, Aprison had demonstrated that changes in levels of a specific neurotransmitter (serotonin) in the brain could be correlated with observable change in the behavior of an animal (pecking or lever pressing for food), an important finding in the expanding efforts to understand the role of neurotransmitters. He had not demonstrated the role of serotonin in depression. The role of neurotransmitters, including serotonin, in major depression and antidepressant medication effects is still a subject of research and is not fully understood even now.

Research continued in Aprison's group with other neurotransmitters and their effects on behavior of laboratory animals. Rats were trained to receive food by lever pressing. In later sessions, foot shock was preceded by white noise when rats started to press the lever. Rats showed observable distress (urination and defecation) with the noxious stimulus of foot shock and did not press the lever for food. Finally, if the noise alone without foot shock occurred, rats would not press the lever for food. Brain acetylcholine was increased in these animals whose behavior had been suppressed as compared with controls, another demonstration of the relation of levels of a neurotransmitter in brain to an animal's behavior.[5] Another example occurred with experiment in GABA and defense response.

GABA and the Defense Reaction

Other studies involved the "calming" neurotransmitter GABA and the "defense reaction" —increase in heart rate and blood pressure with electrical stimulation of the hypothalamus in the brain. Microinjections to the hypothalamus of rats included a GABA blocking drug or a GABA simulating drug. These drugs had opposite effects on the defense response: GABA blockade increased the defense response; stimulation of GABA decreased the symptoms of the defense reaction. These experiments delineated a discrete area of the hypothalamus in which GABA appeared to inhibit the defense response.[6] GABA is important in the actions of anti-anxiety medications and alcohol. Incidentally, both these medications and alcohol are potentially addicting, and GABA is thought to play a role in addictions as well.

More landmark research about neurotransmitters occurred at the Institute of Psychiatric Research when Robert Werman, MD, joined Aprison in 1961. After completing residency in neurology at Mount Sinai Hospital in New York, Werman was a fellow in neurophysiology in the laboratory of Harry Grundfest at Columbia University. Werman later completed a fellowship at the laboratory of Alan Lloyd Hodgkin, soon to be a Nobel Prize winner, in Cambridge, England. Werman and Aprison were the first to demonstrate that the amino acid glycine is an *inhibitory* neurotransmitter in the central nervous system.[7] In other words, glycine blocks the transmission of electrical activity from one neuron to the next rather than enhancing it as do serotonin and norepinephrine.

When Aprison and Werman began their work with glycine, techniques had become available using tiny micropipettes and microelectrodes to measure amounts of neurotransmitters released by single presynaptic cells in living animals and to record the resulting electrical responses in postsynaptic cells. Based on their own work, *they established criteria for proposing a substance as a neurotransmitter: 1) the presence of the compound in the nerve ending of the presynaptic neuron, 2) release of the compound into the synapse, and 3) after attachment to a specific receptor on the postsynaptic neuron stimulation (or inhibition) of an electrical response in the postsynaptic neuron.* They had chosen the lumbosacral region of the cat spinal cord because it had been well studied, and it provided a suitable preparation for their neurochemical/neurophysiological studies. They studied specific areas of the spinal cord where glycine is located, evaluated the role of glycine containing neurons, and demonstrated glycine inhibition of nerve activity.[8]

Theirs and other laboratories were studying the putative brain neurotransmitters acetylcholine, serotonin, norepinephrine, dopamine, glutamate, GABA, and glycine. Many of the neurotransmitters they studied have subsequently been shown to be of importance in the brain and more recently important in the neurochemistry of psychiatric disorders and the pharmacology of medications to treat them. Dopamine and glutamate are thought to be important in schizophrenia and for antipsychotic medicines. Glycine, an inhibitory neurotransmitter, modifies the action at one of the glutamate receptors (NMDA) and has been studied for possible relevance to the treatment of schizophrenia.

Dopamine plays a major role in alcoholism and addiction. Serotonin and norepinephrine are involved with mood disorders. In recognition of his pioneering work studying the role of neurotransmitters in behavior, Aprison received the Gold Medal Award from the Society for Biological Psychiatry and the title of Distinguished Professor from Indiana University, its highest academic honor.

Nurnberger, who had recruited the scientists to the institute, given enthusiastic support to them, and refereed any internecine spats, retired from the chairmanship of the Department of Psychiatry and the directorship of the institute in 1974 but continued on the psychiatry faculty. As one of the leading pioneers of the biological psychiatry movement in the United States, Nurnberger also received the title of Distinguished Professor from Indiana University.

The Institute of Psychiatric Research went through a period of frequent changes in administration for the next few years. James Simmons, MD, a child psychiatrist, was appointed acting chairman of the Department of Psychiatry, and Aprison became director of the institute. In 1975 Hugh Hendrie, MB, ChB, DSc, a native of Scotland, came from the Lafayette Clinic and Wayne State University in Detroit to be chairman of the Department of Psychiatry at Indiana University School of Medicine and executive director of the institute. In 1978 Aprison stepped down as director and Hendrie assumed that position. Hendrie participated in Aprison and Hingtgen's work with antidepressants. Translating laboratory animal studies into potential benefit for patients, they examined the possible role of serotonin in patients with mood disorders, schizophrenia, and anxiety disorders.[9] One way of estimating brain chemicals in living patients is by studying blood levels of those chemicals. Hendrie was involved in clinical studies of the amino acids that act as brain neurotransmitters in blood plasma of depressed and normal individuals.[10] He researched a number of other blood components in psychiatric patients and studied dosage and blood levels of psychotropic medications. He also published articles about the latest findings in psychiatry in the *Journal of the Indiana State Medical Association* for the education of physicians throughout the state.

In one study in 1966 Hendrie collaborated with Joyce Small at Larue Carter Hospital in studies of the effects of lithium, the first effective medication used to treat bipolar disorder.[11] Lithium in liquid solution is an ion, or electrically charged atom, and affects transport of other ions such as sodium, potassium, and calcium ions across membranes including nerve membranes in the production of electrical current. Hendrie and Small measured transport of the amino acids choline and glycine across red blood cell membranes as a mirror of transport across nerve membranes. Working with neurochemist Philip Shea and using rigorous controls, they measured choline and glycine in red blood cells from patients with affective (mood) disorders. Blood samples from normal individuals who had never had lithium, patients with depression or mania who had not had lithium, and other psychiatric patients who had not had lithium were compared with patients with mood disorders who were taking lithium. Red blood cell and plasma choline and red blood cell glycine were increased only in the last group—in other words, the effect on the transport of the amino acids choline and glycine across cell membrane was due to lithium and not to psychiatric illness. Thus, altering membrane transport was one of the actions of lithium. Membrane transport is increasingly being looked at as relevant to mood disorders.

It was during Hendrie's tenure (1975–2000) that a multidepartmental program in the neurosciences was established. Aprison had suggested such a program to medical school dean Steven Beering, who supported it enthusiastically. Aprison had some disagreements about setting up the program, so Hendrie, as chairman of the Department of Psychiatry, appointed Hingtgen as director of the medical neurobiology program. Hendrie and Hingtgen went to the Indiana Higher Education Commission and convinced them of its importance. The commission approved it but with no financial support. The program received major funding and administrative support from the Institute of Psychiatric Research and the Department of Psychiatry and offered master's and doctoral degrees in medical neurobiology. In addition to psychiatry faculty, other participants were recruited from the departments of biochemistry, physiology, medical genetics, anatomy, and pharmacology in the School of Medicine and the departments of biology and psychology of the Purdue School of Science at Indiana University–Purdue University Indianapolis (IUPUI), of which the Indiana University School of Medicine is a part.

Hingtgen, the first director of the program from 1984 until

his retirement in 2000, was succeeded by neurochemist Jay Simon from 2000 to 2010. Their administration and teaching as well as "diplomacy, sweat, and tears" paid off. By the fiftieth anniversary of the institute in 2007, the medical neurobiology program had awarded ten master's degrees and fifty-two doctoral degrees (including eight MD/PhD graduates) and had attracted more than one hundred postdoctoral students from around the world. These students joined faculty in publishing papers in scientific journals as well as dozens of chapters and books—about three thousand publications of institute staff by the end of the first decade of the twenty-first century. In addition the institute and the Department of Psychiatry established an International Symposium on Neuronal Control of Bodily Function. The first meeting had representatives from six countries among its 150 participants and was held in Indianapolis. Subsequent meetings were held in Germany, St. Louis, and California as well as again in Indianapolis. A volume was published annually of the proceedings of the meeting for each of the seven years it was held.[12]

In 1986 Hendrie gave up the directorship of the institute but continued as chairman of the Department of Psychiatry and continued research that would become outstanding in its field—studies of Alzheimer's disease and other dementias in older adults in different cultures around the world. During subsequent years he began international studies, in Canada with Caucasians and Cree Indians, in Jamaica with people of African descent, and in China. He established collaboration with psychiatrists in Nigeria, comparing patients there and African Americans in Indianapolis. The studies evaluate environmental risk factors for Alzheimer's disease such as cardiovascular disease and blood lipoproteins that would be potentially modifiable and thus beneficial in treatment and prevention.

Dementias are characterized by memory loss and loss of intellectual function. There are numerous causes. Alzheimer's dementia involves the gradual loss of memory, thinking, and learning. It usually begins after age sixty-five but might begin before that age. There might or might not be behavioral changes (e.g., agitation, getting lost even in familiar settings). There are disturbances of language, motor function, or ability to plan and organize activities. Although there are characteristic changes in the brain at autopsy, researchers are only beginning to discover techniques for detecting these with certainty in living patients early in the disease.

Hendrie began collaboration in the 1990s with molecular neurobiologist Debomoy Lahiri, PhD, at the institute to study DNA from blood cells in order to determine genes possibly associated with Alzheimer's disease (AD) in the various populations of individuals with the disorder. A particular gene associated with the formation of apolipoprotein E is strongly associated with late-onset Alzheimer's disease in Caucasian populations. Their studies indicated that it is only a weak risk factor in African Americans and not at all in black Nigerians. The prevalence of AD is lower in black Nigerians than in African Americans. Studies of reactions of Nigerian patients' blood cells subjected to chemical tests that damage DNA indicated less reaction than had been seen in similar tests in Caucasians.[13] Most diseases in medicine, including those in psychiatry, appear to be multifactorial, or have multiple factors involved in their causation—a number of genes and a number of environmental factors. These studies bear that out: factors involved in Alzheimer's dementia seem to be different in two ethnic groups.

As part of the World Health Organization Age-Associated Dementias Project, Hendrie developed clinical psychiatric assessment instruments that could be used internationally. He was involved in establishing the Indiana University Center for Aging Research and, in 2000, received the John W. Ryan Award for distinguished contributions to international programs and studies. Hendrie retired as chairman of the Department of Psychiatry in 2000 but continued his research with dementias in older adults. In 2010 he was named to the National Advisory Council on Aging.[14]

Lahiri's research has demonstrated that the course of Alzheimer's disease likely begins early in life and continues over time as environmental stresses occur and epigenetic mechanisms become involved. Epigenetic mechanisms are heritable changes in the chemistry of DNA that influence gene expression without changing the sequence of DNA (see below). Ultimately, genes themselves, their expression now modified by many factors, produce the brain abnormalities of the disorder: beta-amyloid plaques outside neurons and neurofibrilary tangles within neurons. Lahiri and his colleagues studied monkeys administered lead in infancy. Lead is known to be toxic to brains of infants and children. In old age, brains of the monkeys given lead as infants showed increased beta-amyloid precursor protein (APP) and other factors related to formation of the beta-amyloid plaques of Alzheimer's disease. Chemical changes such as methylation of the DNA nucleic acid constituent, cytosine, and oxidation of the nucleic acid, guanosine, also affect gene expression.[15] This model is referred to as the LEARn (Latent Early-life Associated Regulation) model. Stressors during life might include such things as head trauma, poor diet, reduced exercise or even general changes in how some genes affect body chemistry.[16] The ultimate goal of understanding the molecular neurobiology of Alzheimer's is elucidating the causes and successful treatment of the disorder. In addition to over two hundred scientific papers and chapters Lahiri has published in this area, he is founder and editor-in-chief of two major journals, *Current Alzheimer Research* and *Current Aging Science.*

In 1986 Dr. John I. Nurnberger, Jr. came from the National Institute of Mental Health to be director of the Institute of Psychiatric Research thirty years after his father had opened the institute. John Jr. had first come to Indianapolis as a young boy when his family moved from Connecticut so that his father could chair the Department of Psychiatry and the institute. He subsequently received his MD and PhD from Indiana University. He continued the philosophy of the institute initiated from the beginning with emphasis on academic freedom for scientists from many disciplines to pursue their own research interests. His interest and expertise is in the genetics of psychiatric disorders, and he is recognized internationally as a leading scientist in this area. He is coordinator of a national study on the genetics of bipolar disorder and has been centrally involved in the Collaborative Study on the Genetics of Alcoholism (COGA) project, a multisite study of the genetics of alcoholism.

Study of inherited factors in disease has been greatly enhanced by the development of molecular biology and mapping of the human genome. Earlier in the twentieth century, family studies had indicated that most psychiatric disorders, like most medical disorders, run in families whether or not affected individuals share the same environment. Adoption studies show that children are more likely to have the diseases of biological parents than of adoptive parents. Twin studies show that an identical twin is more likely to have an illness that his or her twin has than a fraternal (non-identical) twin. In other words, the more alike individuals are genetically, the more likely they are to have the same diseases.

Genes, Chromosomes, and Heredity

There are twenty-three pairs of chromosomes in each human cell, one of each pair from the mother and the other from the father. Twenty-two pairs each have similar chromosomes; one pair consists of an X and a Y chromosome in males and two X chromosomes in females. Each gene has a specific location on a specific chromosome and a mate ("allele") on the other chromosome of the pair; they are the functional units of heredity and direct the formation of cells and their constituents. Genes are made of DNA (deoxyribonucleic acid). DNA consists of the nucleic acids cytosine, adenine, guanosine, and tyrosine, usually referred to by the first letters of their names: C, A, G, and T. Each nucleic acid is attached to a sugar molecule and a phosphate molecule. A nucleic acid plus a sugar is called a nucleoside. When a phosphate is added, the compound is called a nucleotide. Chromosomes are double strands of DNA twisted into spirals (the "double helix"). The sugars and phosphates form the strands, and two nucleic acids (A + T or G + C) connect each pair of sugar/phosphate in the two strands. There are many nucleotides in each gene, and there are other nucleotides on chromosomes that serve functions such as "switching" specific genes on or off or forming cut-off points for genes in the transfer from DNA to messenger RNA (mRNA) to RNA (ribonucleic acid). Genes pass information to RNA molecules that ultimately bring about the formation of proteins, which have multiple functions throughout the body. Some proteins become building blocks for body tissues, and others make up the enzymes that facilitate the chemical reactions of the body. There are almost three billion nucleotides in the human genome. There are about 23,000 genes that code proteins.

[See illustration p. 143]

Now, the very molecules of inheritance can be studied. Chromosomes in the nucleus at the center of each cell carry the chemical information (strings of genes) to pass on inherited traits. Genome wide association studies (GWAS) compare all the genes of individuals (genomes) with a particular illness to those of individuals who do not have the illness. Abnormalities found frequently in individuals with the illness and not in those who do not have the illness are interpreted as likely related to the illness. The abnormalities that occur include SNPs ("snips," or single nucleotide polymorphisms), single positions where the chromosome carries a different nucleic acid than usual; in other words, the arrangement of C, A, G, or T is "misspelled." Another type of abnormality is CNVs (copy number variants), where a segment of DNA has been duplicated or deleted.

Psychiatric diagnoses, including those we discuss in this and the following chapters, are defined in the Diagnostic and Statistical Manual of Mental Disorders of the American Psychiatric Association, now in its fourth edition (DSM-IV). Definitions involve *groups* of symptoms that occur together and have a common outcome (e.g., get well, fluctuate, prove fatal). As an example, "depression" refers to a mood common to everyone at one time or another. Major depressive disorder refers to an inherited, neurochemical disorder in which the depressed mood is accompanied by changes in sleeping, eating, and activity level; difficulty concentrating; hopelessness; and suicidal thoughts. In other words, ordinary depression is different from major depressive disorder because the latter is a *group* of symptoms representing differences in brain chemistry and genetics. These types of diagnoses have been studied extensively since the nineteenth century. The categories we will discuss are similar to those used by Edenharter and Bahr a century ago. Diagnostic criteria are constantly being fine-tuned as new genetic, neurochemical, psychological, and sociological data become available.

An example of the value of carefully defined diagnoses is autism, which is recognized much more frequently now than in the past. Research has delineated a number of autism spectrum disorders that have some similar characteristics. Marian DeMyer's work, discussed previously, included careful research to determine that autism is not caused by parenting practices. A large autism clinic, the Christian Sarkine Center at James Whitcomb Riley Hospital for Children on the medical school campus, was set up in 1997 when Christopher McDougle, MD, came from the Yale Child Study Center to be director of the Section of Child and Adolescent Psychiatry at Indiana University School of Medicine. His area of expertise is the neurobiology and psychopharmacology of childhood developmental disorders, especially autism and mental retardation. He instituted a unit for research on pediatric psychopharmacology where studies of multiple medications in autism have been carried out. He has commented on the careful use of different medications for the various symptoms of autism, noting the importance of avoiding medicines that actually make symptoms worse. Some symptoms characteristic of autism, for example repetitive behaviors, might actually provide some relief for patients. Choice of whether to prescribe medications requires understanding of the symptoms and their consequences in the individual patient.[17] McDougle became chairman of the Department of Psychiatry in 2000. His work with autism fit well with developing studies at the institute on the genetics of psychiatric disorders. He left to accept a position at Harvard in 2011.

Autism spectrum disorders, including infantile autism and related disorders with similar symptoms, are characterized by impaired social interaction and communication with others and unusual and often repetitive behaviors that begin early in life. Intelligence varies among these individuals. Twin and family studies have favored genetic etiology. About 5 to 15 percent have abnormalities in one gene, rare occurrences in the general population.[18] Nurnberger Jr. and McDougle are part of the Autism Genome Project Consortium, a multisite, multinational group of researchers who have studied individuals with autism at each site. Nurnberger is a lead investigator and a leader in the design and analysis of the study. The consortium has joined with other groups studying autism to provide data about a large number of patients—far more than would be available at any one center. These investigations have identified a SNP on chromosome 5 that is significantly associated with autism and a nearby gene whose expression is reduced in patients with autism. It is related to development of the nervous system in the embryo. Other genes possibly related to autism also have been identified.[19]

When CNVs were studied, it was found that some individuals with autism have multiple abnormalities of this type, even more than had been discovered by earlier methods, especially at locations already implicated in other studies as related to autism. Some of the CNVs disrupted genes involved in cellular proliferation and motility and an enzyme involved in electrical transmission in nerves.

The genetics of autism spectrum disorders is complicated. Many rare single genes can cause similar clinical symptoms. Sometimes there are multiple genetic abnormalities. Most of these genetic abnormalities appear related to genes controlling the development of the nervous system. The multiplicity of genetic abnormalities is consistent with the observation that different patients appear to have different levels and types of disability.[20]

Efforts to learn more about the chemistry and genetics of autism spectrum disorders are focused on the goal of providing better medications and other treatments, tailored to the abilities of each patient. Techniques unavailable to DeMyer are now extending the search for answers to autism. Investigators in the Autism Genome Project are looking at "a whole host of candidate genes for autism . . . in larger samples to see what their prevalence is and how much of a role each of these may play in the genetic predisposition to autism . . . These would be particularly useful as a diagnostic test or as part of a screening panel that persons with autism might receive."[21]

Schizophrenia is a chronic, debilitating disease, often beginning in adolescence. As has been discussed in earlier chapters, it is characterized by psychosis (hallucinations, delusions, bizarre behavior) as well as disorganized speech sometimes to the point of incoherence, grossly disorganized behavior, and "negative" symptoms such as inappropriate emotional responses and poor motivation. Functioning at work or school, interpersonal relationships, and self-care deteriorate.[22] Schizophrenia has been classically defined as a disorder of thinking ("thought disorder"), in contrast to bipolar disorder, a mood disorder ("affective disorder").

Among studies in humans with schizophrenia were studies of sleep patterns carried out with patients at the Roudebush VA Medical Center on the medical school campus by Aimee Mayeda, MD, who is interested in studying circadian (day/night) rhythms in patients. Most subjects were in day treatment and had been carefully diagnosed with schizophrenia or schizoaffective disorder (schizophrenia-like illness with many mood symptoms) using standard criteria. They had not had hospitalizations or medication changes for one month. Activity was measured by a small instrument on the non-dominant wrist. Sleep was rated by each subject on the seven subscales of the Pittsburgh Sleep Quality Index (PSI). Charts were reviewed and research staff assessed clinical symptoms. Analyses of data indicated that poor sleep quality predicted low quality of life and reduced preference for positive reappraisal when faced with a stressor. Poor sleep might play a role in sustaining poor quality of life in individuals with schizophrenia.[23] On the other hand, enhancing sleep might be a useful addition to treatment.

A great deal of research around the world has suggested that individuals suffering from schizophrenia have deficits in information processing, including perception of time. In a study carried out by Anantha Shekhar of the Institute of Psychiatric Research with psychologists at Indiana University and involving thirty-two individuals with schizophrenia and thirty-one non-psychiatrically ill controls, subjects were asked to tap their fingers to computer-generated repetitive tones and to continue tapping after the tones stopped. Those with schizophrenia exhibited significantly faster tapping and greater variability in tapping both with and without tones consistent with deficits in time perception and time reproduction.[24]

Shekhar and colleagues also participated in a multisite study of "sensory gating" in schizophrenia. Not only do individuals with schizophrenia misperceive external happenings but they also perceive "too much"; that is, they are unable to filter out irrelevant information. EEGs measured during auditory stimuli (see Chapter 8) show responses of brain waves that indicate whether the individual being tested is responding to salient stimuli. Schizophrenia patients showed poorer ability to distinguish salient stimuli as compared to control subjects.[25]

Psychiatrist R. Andrew Chambers, MD, has focused his research on dual diagnoses: the presence of both a psychiatric disorder and a substance use disorder (alcoholism, addiction) in the same individual. He has devised an animal model of schizophrenia by making ventral hippocampal lesions in neonatal rats (NVHL). This damages a part of the brain that also has deficits in patients with schizophrenia. When these rats self-administered cocaine, addiction was more likely than in sham-operated controls self-administering cocaine.[26] In other experiments, in which NVHL rats or sham-operated rats were given cocaine or saline injections for five days, the greatest effects were seen in NVHL animals given cocaine—there was hypoactivation of the prefrontal cortical ("executive," higher level) areas and hyperactivation of specific subcortical ("emotional," lower level) areas. The findings suggest that having a psychiatric disorder (in this case an animal model of schizophrenia) compounds the reaction to addicting drugs.[27] A serious problem clinically is that individuals with schizophrenia and other serious psychiatric disorders often use addicting substances rather than their prescribed medications, to their detriment. These kinds of research are a beginning toward better understanding, and hopefully treating, that situation.

The Institute of Psychiatric Research continues the expansion of research into new frontiers by direct examination of animal brain, development of animal models that hopefully mimic human disorders, study of social settings in which disease occurred, study of the human brain via neuroimaging, and study of the human genome as related to psychiatric disorders.

General Reference

E. Passarge, *Color Atlas of Genetics*, 3rd ed. (New York: Thieme, 2007).

Notes

1. M. H. Aprison and J. N. Hingtgen, "Serotonin and Behavior: A Brief Summary," *Federation Proceedings* 31 (1972): 121–29.
2. J. N. Hingtgen, H. C. Hendrie, and M. H. Aprison, "Postsynaptic Serotonergic Blockade Following Chronic Antidepressive Treatment with Trazodone in an Animal Model of Depression," *Pharmacology Biochemistry and Behavior* 20 (1984): 425–28.
3. E. A. Engleman, J. M. Murphy, F. C. Zhou, M. H. Aprison, and J. N. Hingtgen, "Operant Response Suppression Induced with Systemic Administration of 5-Hydroxytryptophan is Centrally Mediated," *Pharmacology Biochemistry and Behavior* 52 (1995): 525–29.
4. M. H. Aprison and J. N. Hingtgen, "A Neurochemist's Perspective on Human Depression and Stress," in *Affective Disorders: Perspectives on Basic Research and Clinical Practice*, ed. T. Kariya and M. Nakagawara (New York: Brunner/Mazel, Inc., 1993), 3–25.
5. J. N. Hingtgen, J. E. Smith, P. A. Shea, M. H. Aprison, and T. M. Gaff, "Cholinergic Changes During Conditioned Suppression in Rats," *Science* 193 (1976): 332–34.

6. A. Shekhar, J. N. Hingtgen, and J. A. DiMicco, "Selective Enhancement of Shock Avoidance Responding Elicited by GABA Blockade in the Posterior Hypothalamus of Rats," *Brain Research* 420 (1987): 118–28.
7. R. Werman, R. A. Davidoff, and M. H. Aprison, "Inhibitory Action of Glycine on Spinal Neurons in the Cat," *Journal of Neurophysiology* 31 (1968): 81–95.
8. M. H. Aprison and R. Werman, "A Combined Neurochemical and Neurophysiological Approach to Identification of Central Nervous System Transmitters," *Neuroscience Research* 1 (1968): 143–74.
9. H. C. Hendrie, J. N. Hingtgen, and M. H. Aprison, "The Role of Serotonin in Affective Disorders, Schizophrenia and Anxiety Disorders," in *Neurobiological Approaches to Human Disease*, ed. D. Hellhammer, I. Florin, and H. Weiner (Toronto: Hans Huber, 1988), 29–43.
10. M. K. DeMyer, P. A. Shea, H. C. Hendrie, and N. N. Yoshimura, "Plasma Tryptophan and Five Other Amino Acids in Depressed and Normal Subjects," *Archives of General Psychiatry* 38 (1981): 642–46.
11. P. A. Shea, J. G. Small, H. C. Hendrie, "Elevation of Choline and Glycine in Red Blood Cells of Psychiatric Patients Due to Lithium Transport," *Biological Psychiatry* 16 (1981): 825–30.
12. J. N. Hingtgen, "The Institute of Psychiatric Research of the Department of Psychiatry and the Indiana University School of Medicine: The Past Prepares for the Future (1956–2007)." Unpublished.
13. D. K. Lahiri, Y. Xu, J. Klaunig, O. Balyewu, A. Ogunniyi, K. Hall, H. Hendrie, and A. Sahota, "Effect of Oxidative Stress on DNA Damage and Beta-Amyloid Precursor Proteins in Lymphoblastoid Cell Lines from a Nigerian Population," *Annals of the New York Academy of Sciences* 893 (1999): 331–36.
14. Newscenter.iupui.edu/4579/Hugh-C-Hendrie.
15. N. H. Zawia, D. K. Lahiri, and F. Cardozo-Pelaez, "Epigenetics, Oxidative Stress and Alzheimer's Disease," *Free Radical Biology and Medicine* 46 (2009): 1241–48.
16. D. K. Lahiri and B. Maloney, "The LEARn (Latent Early-life Associated Regulation) Model Integrates Environmental Risk Factors and the Developmental Basis of Alzheimer's Disease, and Proposes Remedial Steps," *Experimental Gerontology* 45 (2010): 291–96.
17. C. McDougle, presentation at 2010 American Psychiatric Association annual meeting: J. Yan, "Autism Drug Choice Usually Matter of Trial and Error," *Psychiatric News*, July 18, 2010, p. 20.
18. D. Pinto, et al., "Functional Impact of Global Rare Copy Number Variation in Autism Spectrum Disorders," *Nature* 466 (2010), published online at http://www.nature.com/nature/journal/v466/n7304/full/nature09146.html.
19. L. A. Weiss, et al., "A Genome-Wide Linkage and Association Scan Reveals Novel Loci for Autism," *Nature* 461 (2009): 802–08.
20. Ibid.

21. J. I. Nurnberger, Jr., "Autism Research Advances," *Indianapolis Star*, July 18, 2010.
22. *Diagnostic and Statistical Manual of Mental Disorders*, 4th ed, text revision, (Washington, DC: American Psychiatric Association, 2000), 312.
23. J. R. Hofstetter, P. H. Lysaker, and Aimee R. Mayeda, "Quality of Sleep in Patients with Schizophrenia is Associated with Quality of Life and Coping," *BMC Psychiatry* 5 (2005): 13.
24. C. A. Carroll, B. F. O'Donnell, A. Shekhar, and W. P. Hetrick, "Timing Dysfunctions in Schizophrenia as Measured by a Repetitive Finger Tapping Task," *Brain and Cognition* 71 (2009): 345–53.
25. C. A. Brenner, et al., "Event-related Potential Abnormalities in Schizophrenia: A Failure to 'Gate In' Salient Information?," *Schizophrenia Research* 113 (2009): 332–39.
26. R. A. Chambers, "Animal Modeling and Neurocircuitry of Dual Diagnosis," *Journal of Dual Diagnosis* 3 (2007): 19–29.
27. R. A. Chambers, A. M. Sentir, S. K. Conroy, W. A. Truitt, and A. Shekhar, "Cortical-striatal Integration of Cocaine History and Prefrontal Dysfunction in Animal Modeling of Dual Diagnosis," *Biological Psychiatry* 67 (2010): 788–92.

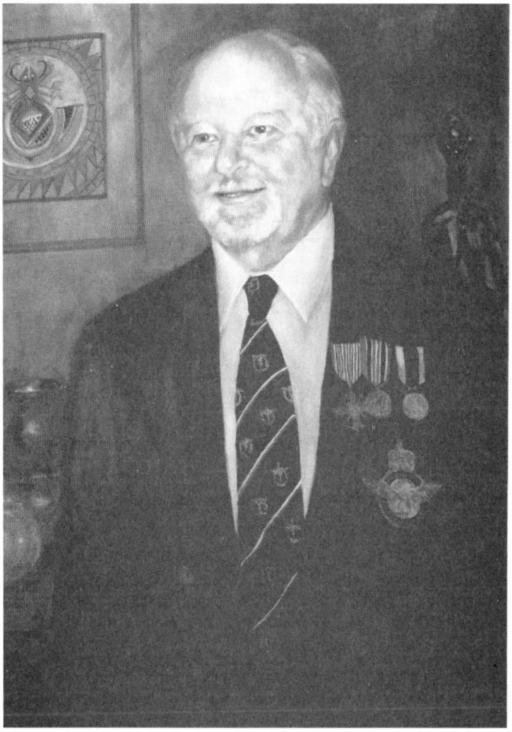

Dr. Hanus Grosz was a clinical researcher who studied anxiety disorders and addictions.

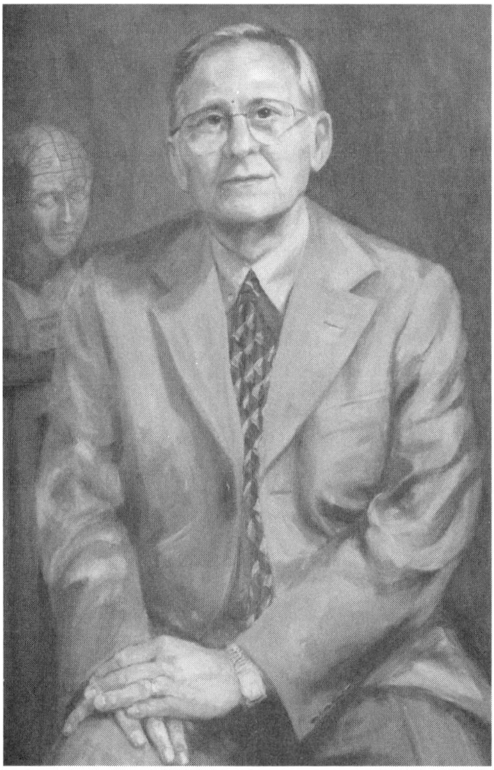

Dr. Joseph Hingtgen designed, organized, and became first director of the multidisciplinary Indiana University Neurobiology Graduate Program.

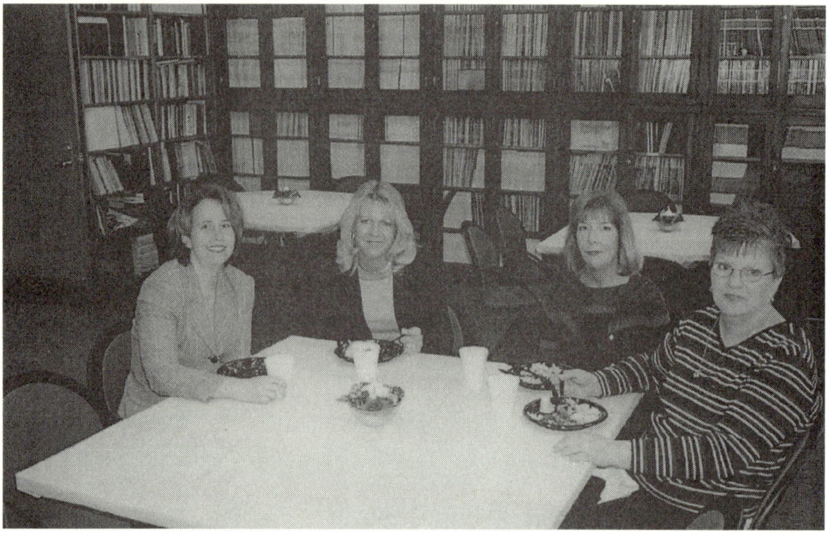

IPR Library, staff members, important members of the Institute's research team, 2000, are(l-r) Jennifer Mullet, Marla Reider, Carrie Fisher, and Patti Warnock.

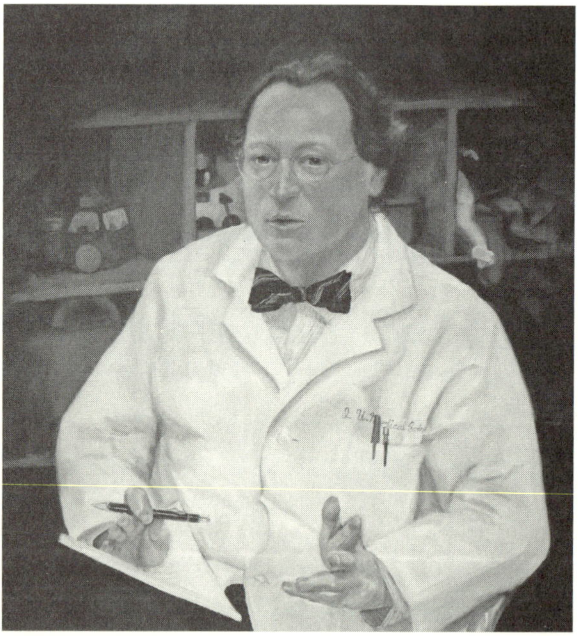

Dr. Christopher McDougle, whose selection as a Richter Scholar in Child Psychiatry as a medical student at Indiana University led to a career in research and treatment of autism, as well as, ultimately, chairmanship of the Department of Psychiatry.

7
Two Women

Larue Carter Hospital III

Women were entering professions in greater numbers and assuming more important roles in academia and in health care administration as the second half of the twentieth century progressed. Larue Carter Memorial Hospital participated in this trend with two very capable women superintendents who served consecutively and helped to advance both the science and the social climate for care of the mentally ill. It is well to consider their special contributions.

A dedicated teacher and an advocate for the chronically mentally ill, Clare M. Assue, MD, was born in New York City in 1922 and later graduated from Hunter College in that city. She received her medical training at Howard University in Washington, DC. Assue first came to Larue Carter Hospital in 1958, and in 1980 she became the first African American woman to serve as superintendent of any state psychiatric hospital in the U.S.[1]

Assue was a professor of psychiatry at Indiana University School of Medicine, director of psychiatry residency training, and coordinator of the undergraduate [medical student] curriculum committee in psychiatry. In addition, she was a consultant at Midtown Mental Health Center and Roudebush Veterans Affairs Hospital on the medical school campus. Even now, mention of her name to anyone who experienced her teaching elicits spontaneous praise for her abilities as a mentor. She not only became involved in education at the medical school, but she also participated on boards of an elementary school and a secondary school in the community as well as on a judicial study commission for the Indiana Juvenile Justice Division. These and other activities led to her being designated a Sagamore of the Wabash, the highest honor awarded by the governor of Indiana.[2]

Speaking to an audience of psychiatrists at a continuing medical educational session, Assue outlined her perspective on the care of the chronically mentally ill. Her lecture was reprinted in a national publication of the American Psychiatric Association.[3] She noted that as outpatients, such individuals were traditionally given fifteen-minute appointments at mental health clinics. "Well, 15 minutes doesn't do very much for very many people . . . and certainly didn't do enough for schizophrenics," she said. "What then does have to be put into play to talk about after-treatment [post-hospitalization] as opposed to a holding or maintenance or supporting operation?" She noted further the importance of an ongoing supportive relationship with either a [professional] person or a [mental health] facility. This has to begin quickly after hospital discharge and evolve into an appropriate relationship. Patients with these lifelong illnesses need at least three to six months with the same therapist or at least several people who "can pick up and really move with the patient." In discussing the interplay of psychosocial and medication treatments, she pointed out that "[y]ou cannot even institute the elements of non-drug management until there is some kind of stable appreciation between the patient, the therapist physician, and the family about the use of medication."

Because antipsychotic medications had been available for more than two decades, it was then known (1980) that there were severe long-term neurological side effects and that treatment failures occurred. These facts were "pushing us more now to use drugs more focally, individually, and thoughtfully." It is important to be flexible about the use of medication. It can't be predicted who needs medication continually, or who needs it only during a psychotic episode—or who needs small doses or who needs large doses all the time. It becomes for the psychiatrist a matter of trial and error and, therefore, becomes important to educate patient and family about the disease process. "It's for you and the patient to identify why he needs drugs, why this particular drug, and how much he is supposed to take," Assue observed.

"I think that the business of education is one of the primary things [in treatment]," she continued. It is important to help the patient to "sort what is normal from what is abnormal in his thinking." The physician can educate the family "to be alert and respond to the patient's behavior, feelings, and perceptions." She discussed various kinds of unhelpful family situations and emphasized the importance of "teaching the patient and family to be able to separate," i.e. the patient needs to lead his own life as much as possible. Most important is the need for "safety, asylum, and care."

With every patient it is important to do a mental status exam and physical examination and to assess psychological and intellectual function as well as vocational skills and aptitudes. Role-playing can be used to help the patient learn to function in society. If he will be unable to work at gainful employment, volunteer work might be useful for a "feeling of adequacy or meaningfulness." If there is to be residential placement, it must be carefully planned. Regular medical care is essential for any patient.

Severely, chronically mentally ill patients are difficult to work with, but Assue insisted that the psychiatrist must be "willing to try with each patient." Assue's philosophy of the care of such patients represents the best of care today: treatment tailored to the individual patient; involvement of patient and family in treatment planning, educating both patient and family about the illness and its treatment; and flexibility in finding the best combination of resources for each individual patient. Although we are beginning to be able to select a particular medication for a particular patient, the necessity remains for thoughtful trial and error.

Assue was very excited about the potential for her new position at Carter Hospital upon her appointment as superintendent. She had always been a great supporter of her predecessor, Donald Moore, but she was also pragmatic to a fault. If Moore was "out," and she was "in," she would make the most of the opportunity this presented. But very shortly after her appointment to her new duties, tragedy struck her family. Her husband, Frank Brown, also a physician, was diagnosed with lung cancer. As the disease ravaged his health, it also had a huge effect on Assue. Like most wives of that era, she was not only the major, but pretty much the only, caretaker of the sick within her home. The effort of tending to her ailing husband clearly sapped a lot of her own energy. As forceful and hard working as Assue was, few probably noticed the change that came over her work once her husband was diagnosed. But Assistant Superintendent Iver Small knew her well, and he could see how much this extra burden, willing as she was to take it on, was weighing upon her.

Her husband's illness ultimately came to the usual end at that time, and he passed away after some four years of declining health. Assue did some grieving and then began to get back to the business of making Carter Hospital the best treatment, research, and learning institution it could be. It was not long, however, before she herself was diagnosed with the same condition that had just taken her husband's life. For the next five years, Assue continued to struggle to make her vision for Carter Hospital into a reality, but the disease was stronger even than this little whirlwind of a teacher and administrator. Again, Small was there, and he recalls wondering how she ever made it back from the hospitalizations required from time to time to try to slow the inevitable tide of her illness. When he visited her on one occasion late in her illness, he says she had turned a sickly green color, and he thought, "She'll never make it this time." But the following week, her children brought her into her office, "propped her up in her chair," and she "soldiered on" for several more months. Ultimately her poor health necessitated her resignation as superintendent in 1989, and she died not long after, in 1990.

Assue's successor was Diana Haugh, MS, RN, a graduate of the Indiana University School of Nursing who had also earned a master's degree in administration from Indiana University. She was superintendent of Larue Carter Memorial Hospital from 1990 to 2003. Early in her career she had worked for a number of years as a staff nurse on the units at Carter Hospital. She then became associate director of adult surgery at Indiana University Hospital and subsequently was an administrator in the central office of the Indiana Department of Mental Health. Although the first non-physician to serve as superintendent of Carter Hospital, unlike most physicians she had credentials in administration. Her background certainly provided experiences relevant to directing a state psychiatric hospital. Haugh continued the focus on patient care, teaching, and research and established the "recovery" model at Carter Hospital. This model of mental health treatment not only uses all the resources available to assist the patient as described by Assue but also focuses on hope for the future and emphasizes the positive abilities the patient has, not just the illness and its negative consequences.

Haugh grew up on the east side of Indianapolis, the eldest of seven children. Initially, it was her mother who developed an interest in a nursing career, but with children and the responsibilities that a family brings, it never quite happened. By the time she was four years of age, though, young Diana knew she wanted to go into nursing. She has two sisters and a daughter who are also nurses.

A big task facing this superintendent in 1997 was the move of all patients and staff to a different building a couple of miles away from the original Tenth Street facility. The veterans' hospital was moving psychiatric patients and staff from a satellite building on Cold Spring Road to its main medical facility on the medical school campus, leaving its former psychiatric hospital (originally designed as sort of residential facility for housing and treating veterans with tuberculosis) unoccupied. The original Larue Carter Memorial Hospital had become crowded with the 1994 closing of Central State Hospital where Dr. Edenharter had worked. Patients formerly at Central State were now housed at Carter.

A word about that event is in order, since this story has its beginnings and much of its development at Central State Hospital. Central, as it was always called by Indianapolis citizens when they were not calling it "Seven Steeples," situated as it was in Indiana's most intense media center, had long been a target of investigative reporting and exposés about problems with patient care. Since the 1950s Central had been continuing its care of the chronically mentally ill. The huge numbers the hospital had had in previous decades were continually diminishing because of outpatient and quick-turnaround, return-to-society care. Central was seeing a steady stream of outpatient cases; the advent of newer medicines and resultant smaller inpatient population was not sufficient to solve all of the difficulties this aging and often sparsely funded institution experienced. After the deaths of two patients from medicine overdoses, the state put together a panel to review medication policies and procedures at the hospital, which one of the authors, Alan Schmetzer, chaired. His own voice tells that personal story:

> I feel fairly sure looking back on it that the governor at the time, Evan Bayh, would probably have preferred our committee to find that Central State was far past the point at which remedial action would help anything. But we dutifully followed the public charge we were given, and after interviewing multiple staff members and talking with some patients and families, we came up with a list of improvements that we believed would solve the deaths from medicines and overdoses.
>
> Our recommendations worked—no more deaths at the hospital could be attributed to medication overdose. Unfortunately, a flurry of well-publicized deaths from other causes then became the nemesis of Central State Hospital. The hospital staff members were told in no uncertain terms that no more deaths on grounds could occur. When a patient who was supposed to have been on one-to-one observation—that is, to have had a member of the staff with her every minute—drowned while in a bathtub one evening (possibly a suicide, since that was what the one-to-one observation was put in place to prevent) the staff reportedly dried her off, put her nightgown on her, and placed her back in bed before calling the physician on duty to initiate resuscitation. It was clear to the doctor that something was amiss.

An investigation easily turned up the actual chain of events.

Central State Hospital's closure was a foregone conclusion, and it occurred in 1994. Larue Carter Hospital was designated as the place that former Central State employees with sufficient seniority could "bump" more recent hires. Most of the Central State staff members were very long-term state employees, so about half of Carter Hospital's staff were "bumped" from their positions. As many patients as possible were dispersed to various community placements made possible by freed-up dollars previously used to care for them at Central. However, a number could not be released and had to be moved to other state hospitals, with the majority going to Carter Hospital due to its proximity to their families. These were troubled and tumultuous times for mental health care-givers and their patients in Indianapolis.

Carter itself was now overcrowded with the arrival of the additional patients from Central, and due to asbestos in the building, remodeling and enlargement were not options. Haugh had become good friends with the VA administrator, Alice Wood. In one of their conversations, the idea of some sort of "land swap" came up. The VA needed more room for parking and to enlarge its facility to accommodate the people who had been moved from its Cold Spring Road facility. It was also desirous of finding a way to offload the maintenance cost of the old building, which continued despite its having been vacated. Carter needed more room, too, and required more green space—"hospital grounds." Over the years, parking lots—always a huge need at an urban medical school campus—had encroached on the land around the original Larue Carter Hospital. The two women decided that swapping facilities would solve both of their problems. An agreement was written and signed by officials from both the federal government and the state, "leasing" the VA facility for twenty years to the state for the use of Carter Hospital for a lump sum payment of $10,000,000. After twenty years the state would own the facility outright. The agreement also gave the Carter property to the VA, with an expectation that the building would be torn down and replaced with a new parking garage.

But the best-laid plans often go astray. Tearing Carter down proved way too expensive—the asbestos that prevented remodeling also made the demolition of the building a multi-million dollar liability. And no one had taken into account that the land that Carter was built upon actually belonged to Indiana University and not to the state of Indiana directly.

Larue Carter's move was completed before all of these problems could be discovered. Haugh had a huge set of tasks in not only integrating the Central State employees and patients with Carter's, but then moving everyone into a different building about a mile and a half away. Construction of the original VA Cold Spring Road facility had begun in 1933, at the height of a tuberculosis epidemic among the veteran population. After that crisis abated, the building was used for medical patients. Finally the VA's hospital's entire mental health program was moved to the Cold Spring Road building in the late 1970s. During the 1980s, extensive remodeling and a new addition under the leadership of Service Chief John Sullivan, MD, helped make the facility more useful for psychiatric treatment purposes. But the biggest attraction of the move for Haugh was the availability of more than twenty fenced-in acres around the main building. The larger interior space and unencumbered surrounding grounds seemed like a reasonable trade to Haugh and her superiors at the Division of Mental Health.

Carter Hospital was established in its new building when it celebrated its fiftieth anniversary in 2002. In a brochure that accompanied that celebration, Haugh reflected on the role of the hospital in comments reminiscent of Moore's earlier statement that a "hospital is an extension of the community." Haugh wrote, "Healthy communities are those that engage in dialogue and transform themselves through practices to improve health and overall quality of life. Continuing to educate and creating increasingly effective treatments and service delivery for mental illness will go a long way to reduce the stigma of a mental illness. We must be a part of the community dialogue, carry out our tri-fold mission of treatment, teaching and research with resolve, and be open to strategic renewals and continue change."

"As we collaborate and work together to generate new knowledge about the brain, behavior and total health," she continued, "we must participate in translating that knowledge to the service systems, providers and citizens. We are challenged to meet the demands of the future along with our health and social service agencies, policy makers, employers, communities and citizens. Let us move forward together."[4]

Haugh continued to do just that over the next year, but an event was already beginning to unfold that would end her tenure as Carter Hospital's superintendent almost as tragically as the events that had conspired against Assue, although of an entirely different nature.

As a volunteer at Carter Hospital after her retirement from Eli Lilly & Co., Martha Stamper had developed a great fondness for the Carter Hospital Professional Library. The School of Medicine and the rest of the state hospital system relied heavily on Carter to have not only an historical archive of books and journals relating to mental health, but the very latest writings on psychiatric subject matter as well. Haugh and the Department of Psychiatry had collaborated to maintain as much funding for the library as possible, since state legislators did not seem to believe in the importance of such a facility, at least from the standpoint of providing adequate dollars. Stamper was well aware of this struggle, so at her death she left half of her money—and over a half-million dollars—to Carter Hospital to be used "for the library." This windfall would be immensely useful in maintaining the library—*if* it could be used for its donor's intended purpose.

Any money coming to the state, whatever the intended purpose, goes not to a given institution or office, but into the state's "general fund." Haugh knew this only too well, and she could see the money sailing blithely on from her office to fund a bridge in Delaware County or a park in Evansville, also good, useful, and necessary purposes, but not what Stamper had in mind for her donation. So, Haugh placed the check into the hospital safe and began a lengthy (nearly two-year-long) negotiation with state administrators over how the money would actually be used. Eventually, an agreement was reached, and the Stamper Center was created at Carter Hospital, with the money being used to refurbish the library; upgrade the auditorium (and name it for long-time hospital clinician-researchers, Joyce and Iver Small); improve the hospital's internal TV programming system and expand telecommunications capability into the former chapel, now termed the "Board Room;" create two additional conference rooms (the Dewey Room and the Murray Room, housing a veritable library of books donated by William Murray's family); and remodel space that was to be leased to the Indiana Chapter of the National Alliance on Mental Illness (NAMI) for their state offices.

The negotiations finally complete, in 2005, Haugh turned the check over to state officials. She was, unfortunately and as a result of her action in keeping the check, terminated and "sued" by the state over fiscal malfeasance. The claim was that Indiana had lost "thousands of dollars" of interest on the original donation because the check had not been turned over. Immediately local media made the case sound like some sort of "embezzlement," but although the authors do not claim to know all of the facts involved, it would appear to us that, if Haugh had been "guilty" of anything, it would simply be trying to follow a donor's wishes for the use of her money.[5]

Nonetheless, Haugh was now gone from Carter Hospital, and thus ended an era of relative stability for tenures of Carter Hospital superintendents. Assue had continued in spite of personal tragedy to provide excellent patient care and teaching while supporting research. Haugh had weathered very trying political turmoil while focusing on the recovery mode of emphasizing patient strengths.

During the first fifty years of its existence, Carter Hospital had been led by only four superintendents—Drs. Nielsen, Moore, and Assue, and Ms. Haugh. As the subsequent chapters illustrate, there have been about as many superintendents of the hospital over the past five years as during the first fifty.

Notes

1. Funeral Program, Dr. Clare Assue Brown, Trinity Episcopal Church, Indianapolis; obituary, *Indianapolis Star*, August 30, 1990.
2. Ibid.
3. *Psychiatric News* 15 (November 7, 1980): 1.
4. "50 years of Serving Mental Health in Indiana: LARUE D. CARTER MEMORIAL HOSPITAL, 2002, a brochure put out by the hospital.
5. An example of such stories, published by Channel 8 News (WISH-TV) on August 14, 2003: "Psych Hospital—Missing money to be repaid: The former superintendent at Larue Carter Psychiatric Hospital is now agreeing to pay $35,000 to the state for mishandling a half-million-dollar estate gift. Diana Haugh was being sued by the state for $42,000 in lost interest after she failed to deposit the funds. The money was kept secret for two years until state auditors discovered it."

Diana Haugh was a pioneer of the Recovery Model in state institutions, helping patients to focus on their strengths rather than weaknesses and giving them hope.

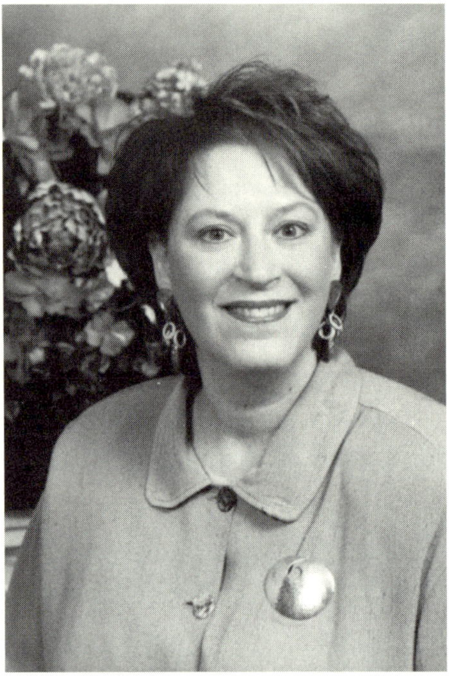

Dr. Clare Assue was the third superintendent at Larue Carter Hospital and the second Director of Residency Training in the Department of Psychiatry, Indiana University School of Medicine. Her dedication to patient care enhanced both roles.

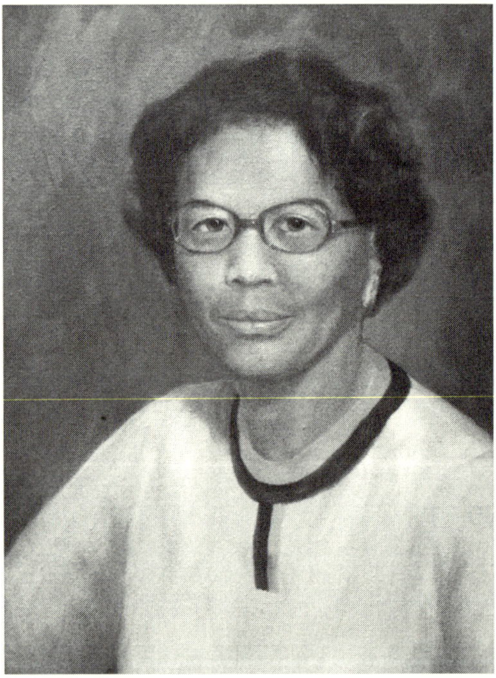

8
Of Rats and Men Under the Influence
Alcoholism and Addiction
The Institute of Psychiatric Research III

"The cure for alcoholism, Doc, would be if you could give me a shot, and then for the rest of my life, I could walk into a bar, have one drink, and leave." This denizen of a Salvation Army mission for alcoholics was absolutely correct. Individuals who use alcohol but not to excess can walk into a bar, have one drink, and leave. Individuals with alcoholism (alcohol dependence) cannot stop at just one drink. Genes have a lot to do with both types of behavior. In the past three decades, genetic studies at the Institute of Psychiatric Research have been identifying how genes play their important role in this debilitating disease.

Alcoholism is one of the most devastating of all disorders, affecting not only the individual but also the family, the workplace, and the community. Spousal abuse, neglect of children, drunk driving that might harm others, poor work performance, and health problems such as damage to the heart, liver, stomach, and brain are just a few of the possible consequences. The man quoted above was in a mission for the destitute—he had no money, having lost any jobs he had; he had no family who would take him in; he was dependent on others' contributions to a nonprofit organization for food and shelter and help getting sober. Achieving sobriety for an individual with alcoholism is one of the most difficult of human tasks. Once achieved, there is a battle to maintain sobriety. Hence, Alcoholics Anonymous and other self-help groups as well as inpatient and outpatient treatment centers provide long-term follow-up with the support of professionals and other individuals, many of whom have themselves conquered their dependence on alcohol.

That genetics can be shown to be a major cause of alcoholism lifts a terrible burden of thousands of years in which victims, the "drunks" of society, were viewed only as weak individuals who lacked moral stamina and character and caused their own problems. Genetic predisposition belies those personally devastating societal views. If alcoholism treatment can continue to be significantly improved, that will be an encouraging promise of the present and the goal of the future. Scientists in Indiana have been devoting themselves to these goals as a new century has unfolded.

Nowhere has collaboration of the Institute of Psychiatric Research with other departments of the School of Medicine been more productive than in efforts to determine causes of, and treatment for, alcoholism. An animal model of alcohol dependence was developed at the Indiana Alcohol Research Center (IARC) on the medical school campus in the 1970s by Ting-Kai Li, MD, in collaboration with Lawrence Lumeng, MD, a graduate of Indiana University School of Medicine and for many years the chief of the Division of Gastroenterology and Hepatology of the Department of Medicine at the medical school. A special visiting lectureship in that division has been named for Lumeng. Li was born in China and, as a young boy, escaped with his family as the Japanese were bombing their hometown in the late 1930s. After a journey across three continents, they came to the United States, where "T-K" graduated from Northwestern University and Harvard Medical School. After twenty years as director of the Indiana Alcohol Research Center, he was appointed director of the National Institute on Alcohol Abuse and Alcoholism of the National Institutes of Health in Bethesda, Maryland. The credentials and dedication of these scientists point to the importance genetic research has gained here as well as elsewhere.

The importance of genetic factors in the response to alcohol was demonstrated by differences in alcohol consumption brought about by animal genetic manipulation (selective breeding).[1] Lumeng and Li took advantage of the fact that, in a strain of inbred rats, there will be a few who drink alcohol when given a choice even though most animals will not choose alcohol. They bred male and female rats that had been demonstrated to drink alcohol even when given other choices. In each subsequent generation, alcohol-preferring rats were selected and bred. After several generations they had established a line of "P" or alcohol-preferring rats. Similarly, they took rats from the original group that demonstrated greatest aversion to alcohol consumption and established a line of "NP" or non-preferring rats. These animal lines have been used worldwide in research about alcoholism.

The public is often curious about the important use of rats in experiments. Clearly their use has been vital in the alcoholism studies. Rats are housed in breeding colonies in medical school animal resource facilities accredited by the Association for Assessment and Accreditation of Laboratory Animal Care. Experimental procedures must be approved by the Institutional Animal Care and Use Committee of the IU School of Medicine in accordance with guidelines of the National Institutes of Health. Rats reach adulthood at ninety days of age and are housed in hanging wire-mesh cages in metal racks. Food and water are available from a water bottle with a stopper holding an angled stainless steel sipper tube and a food hopper attached to the side of each cage. In the case of the alcohol research, alcohol solutions are available through other sipper tubes. Maintaining the breeding colony is a time-consuming task. There have been more than fifty generations of these animals. Experiments must have many controls in order to be sure that what is being measured is, indeed, what the experimenter wants to measure, as will be described below.

The IARC (Lumeng and Li's) group performed a number of experiments to establish that P rats deal with alcohol in the same way humans with alcohol dependence do (i.e., are a good model for alcoholism). P rats voluntarily consume much more alcohol daily than NP rats, resulting in high blood levels of alcohol. P rats will work by pressing a bar to obtain alcohol even if food and water are available. They will work to have alcohol delivered through a gastric tube or directly into the brain, which means that it isn't taste, smell, or caloric value that governs their use of alcohol but rather the pharmacologic effects. The rats develop *tolerance* to the motor impairments of high levels of alcohol (they can hold their liquor without appearing drunk) and *physical dependence* (withdrawal symptoms when high-dose alcohol is stopped), both among the symptoms of alcohol dependence. NP rats show none of these behaviors. Other similar lines were also developed from a different original strain of rats: HAD "high alcohol drinking" and LAD "low alcohol drinking." All of these rats were also compared with an entirely different strain of rats "W" (Wistar) as a control.[2]

People who have alcohol dependence consume much larger quantities of alcohol than others can handle. They are tolerant to these large amounts and ultimately develop withdrawal if they stop drinking—sweating, tremor, nausea, anxiety, agitation, even convulsions or hallucinations. They lose control and drink more and longer than they meant to do. They might try to control drinking by setting time limits or drinking only under certain circumstances, but such efforts are ineffective. They neglect important responsibilities at home, work, or in the community. Some individuals with this disorder are violent to loved ones, friends, or even strangers when under the influence. Initially, they drink alcohol to get "high." As time goes on, they drink to avoid withdrawal symptoms.

Individuals with alcohol dependence who have been abstinent for a period of time and then relapse to drinking again will at first drink more than they did before the period of abstinence. This Alcohol Deprivation Effect was demonstrated in P and HAD lines of alcohol-preferring rats after several months of alcohol exposure and two weeks of deprivation. However, the responses of P rats and HAD lines were different when short periods of deprivation—deprivation for four days, then access to alcohol for four days, repeated for a total of four cycles—were studied. These shorter periods of deprivation and exposure are a model of binge drinking. Both lines of rats showed a one-hour Alcohol Deprivation Effect, with blood alcohol increasing significantly. HAD lines, but not P rats, showed a twenty-four-hour deprivation effect (heavier than usual drinking for twenty-four hours). Thus the differing genetic make-up of P and HAD lines of rats influences the duration of the Alcohol Deprivation Effect after binge drinking. Because there are likely several types of alcoholism in humans, these findings of differences among the animal model groups are useful in helping to define the different types of alcoholism in humans and ultimately to focus on which treatments work best for which patients.[3]

At the Institute of Psychiatric Research, biochemist William McBride, PhD, who had worked with Morris Aprison, now began the neurochemical studies of the IARC "alcoholic" and "nonalcoholic" rats. The work of genes, "gene expression," involves transfer of genetic information from DNA to RNA and ultimately to formation in cells of proteins, which are composed of amino acids. The multitude of proteins in the brain and body include both enzymes that facilitate chemical reactions that would not otherwise occur at body temperature and acidity and structural building blocks for cells and tissues. P and NP rats were studied for protein expression in a part of the brain known to be important in alcoholism and addiction, the nucleus accumbens. Rats were given repeated injections of alcohol into the abdominal cavity (intraperitoneal). Rats were then sacrificed and their brains frozen.

Experimenters used liquid chromatography/ mass spectroscopy, an extremely sensitive and specific method for identifying chemicals, to determine proteins in specific small areas of the brains. Researchers compared P rats injected with saline (controls) to those injected with alcohol and NP rats injected with saline (controls) to those injected with alcohol. Alcohol administration altered expression levels of proteins in both P rats and NP rats. However, the proteins changed were different in the different lines of rats. In NP rats, the proteins increased by alcohol were related to electrical transmission in neurons and transmission across synapses. These changes with initial exposure to alcohol might be related to the low alcohol-drinking characteristics of NP rats and by analogy to humans who do not develop alcoholism even though they drink alcohol. There were fewer protein changes in P rats than in NP rats, but some of them suggested synaptic changes in these rats. In other words, there were synaptic changes in P and NP rats, but the changes were in different proteins.[4]

Li, Lumeng, McBride, and their colleagues found a deficiency of serotonin in P and HAD rats in several brain regions, including the frontal cortex (the "executive" part of the brain) and nucleus accumbens (an area of the brain important in drug and alcohol dependence). Serotonin systems control mood, eating and drinking behavior, and the development of tolerance to alcohol. It will be recalled from previous chapters that serotonin is also implicated in mood disorders. Serotonin also modulates the release of dopamine, a neurotransmitter that has an important role in motor activity, enhancing response to drugs, and reward (pleasurable feelings), i.e., it is important in addiction. P and HAD lines have lower dopamine in the nucleus accumbens. P rats are more sensitive to the release of dopamine in the nucleus accumbens by small doses of alcohol. (They get more "bang for the buck" than NP rats). P rats are more anxious and more sensitive to stressful stimuli, possibly related to changes in GABA neurons. (GABA "calms" responses to stress.) P and NP rates also differed in the presence of the body's own opiod-related (pain-killing) chemicals.[5]

The teams performing surgery on rat brains and administering alcohol to rats via microcannulas (tiny tubes) carefully implanted into specific brain areas demonstrated what brain pathways are important in alcohol dependence. Both P ("alcoholic") rats and W ("non-alcoholic") rats pressed levers to infuse alcohol into the shell, but not into the core, of the nucleus accumbens, indicating that the shell is the structure mediating the reinforcing actions of alcohol. P rats pressed levers for more alcohol than W rats.[6]

McBride and his group, continuing experiments into the twenty-first century, delineated the additional specific areas in the brain that are important in alcohol effects. The dopamine system in the brain that is important in alcohol and drug dependence originates in the ventral tegmental area (VTA) and projects to the nucleus accumbens. Research with blockers of dopamine D2 receptors and of GABAA receptors showed that dopamine neurons in the posterior VTA may be under greater dopamine D2 receptor inhibition, whereas dopamine neurons in the anterior VTA may be under greater GABAA receptor inhibition.[7]

For each neurotransmitter there are several receptors to which it can attach on the various cells it influences. Ethanol intake was lower ("non-alcoholic") in rats with: 1) increased synaptic levels of serotonin or dopamine; 2) activation of the serotonin receptors 5-HT1A or 5-HT2, the dopamine receptors D2 or D3, or the GABAA receptor; or 3) blocking of opioid and 5-HT3 receptors. In other words, more serotonin, dopamine, and GABA activity at certain receptors and less opioid activity were associated with *not* drinking excessively.[8] Blocking of opioid receptors is used in the treatment of alcohol dependence in humans. Psychologist Dena Davidson, PhD, collaborating with researchers at Brown University, studied naltrexone, an opioid blocker, plus psychological treatments in non-treatment-seeking heavy drinkers recruited through newspaper advertisements. Naltrexone was given to these individuals, who also received either motivational enhancement therapy (MET) or broad spectrum treatment (BST), a cognitive behavioral therapy tailored to each patient's specific needs. After twelve weeks of treatment with naltrexone, one-half of each psychotherapy group was continued on naltrexone, and the other half of each group given placebo. The median time to first drink and time to first heavy drinking day were significantly longer for the group receiving naltrexone for twenty-four weeks plus BST than for any other group.[9] Delineating what treatment combinations are most effective is currently of great importance in the treatment of alcoholism as new medications and psychotherapies become available.

In collaboration with the Institute of Psychiatric Research and the Indiana Alcohol Research Center, the Neuropsychology Group in the Department of Neurology at the medical center uses noninvasive brain imaging techniques, fMRI (functional magnetic resonance imaging), and PET (positron emission tomography) to study the response of the brain to alcohol in adult humans who have a variety of drinking patterns Neuropsychologist David Kareken, PhD, uses fMRI, a neuroimaging method that measures oxygen use in the different parts of the brain, thus indicating which parts are most active under different experimental conditions. After priming doses of alcohol, sniffing alcoholic beverage odors increased nucleus accumbens activity. In another study, ten of Davidson's hazardous drinking subjects were given functional magnetic resonance imaging (fMRI) scans. Subjects received intravenously either lactate Ringer's solution (commonly used in intravenous solutions) or lactate Ringer's solution with alcohol. Subjects sniffed non-food odors such as leather, food odors (chocolate or grape), or alcohol. Alcohol intravenously enhanced brain activity only after alcohol odors—not other odors—in orbitofrontal, medial frontal, and precuneus/posterior cingulate regions, all cerebral cortical areas connected to the limbic system in the brain that includes the nucleus accumbens and other areas involved in alcoholism and addiction as well as in mood and emotion.[10]

Another study looked at stress and drinking behavior in alcohol-dependent subjects recruited by Davidson. Like most body/brain reactions, dealing with stress involves a system, not just one structure or chemical. The hypothalamic-pituitary-adrenal (HPA) axis is involved in dealing with stress. The hypothalamus in the brain is the "thermostat" that keeps body functions such as blood pressure and temperature in balance. Among other activities, it sends a hormone (CRF) through blood vessels to the pituitary, the master gland located just below the brain that controls many other body glands. The pituitary, in turn, sends another hormone (ACTH) through the blood circulation to the adrenal glands just above the kidneys in the abdomen. The adrenals then send out the stress hormone, cortisol.

Cortisol was measured in saliva in Davidson's heavy-drinking subjects. In some of the subjects, blood samples were used to assess a gene variant that is associated with the μ-opioid receptor. (The opioid system is the body's own pain-relieving mechanism.

The μ-opioid receptor is also involved in regulating reward, such as pleasure when drinking alcohol, and aversion, such as eating something very bitter.) When this gene is present, the μ-opioid receptor exhibits a blunted response to stress. Stress was induced in these subjects with a psychological test in which the subjects heard a number every three seconds and were required to keep adding the numbers serially. Subjects were studied in two separate sessions, one without stress and the other with the stressful test. With stress there was less salivary cortisol and more alcohol intake compared with the sessions without stress. There was a trend for those with the gene variant to have even less cortisol response and more alcohol intake with stress. These experiments demonstrated some of the genomic and environmental factors that play a part in individuals who drink excessive amounts.[11] In other words, heavy drinkers had a diminished response to stress and at the same time drank more alcohol when stressed. Given these responses, they would not be expected to react effectively to difficult situations. A particular gene related to pain control and reward, the HPA hormonal system, and an environmental stress combined to diminish the performance of a heavy drinker.

Sean O'Connor, MD, a psychiatrist with a background in engineering, works with individuals with alcoholism at the Veterans Affairs Medical Center on the medical school campus and at the Institute of Psychiatric Research. He developed a method of intravenous infusion of alcohol in humans, measuring breath alcohol simultaneously, to maintain constant blood alcohol levels. From these data the brain level of alcohol is calculated and maintained constant. O'Connor, Kareken, and others using this method of alcohol infusion plus PET neuroimaging—positron emission tomography that measures blood flow, and thus activity, in various parts of the brain—found variations from individual to individual in brain dopamine release with alcohol. However, when they used special techniques to observe the area (near the nucleus accumbens) with greatest dopamine release in each individual subject compared with that subject's report of intoxication, there was a correlation of dopamine release and response to alcohol.[12] The neurotransmitter dopamine is important for reward with pleasurable emotions after eating, drinking, sexual activity, and the like. This finding is consistent with the animal studies of lower dopamine in alcohol-preferring rats' brains, i.e., individuals who drink heavily appear to be stimulating dopamine production in their brains, which have lower than normal amounts.

Phenotypes are observable physical traits related to particular genes (e.g., eye color). Physical traits that are not externally visible but are measurable are called endophenotypes, for example the cortisol measured in experiments described above. Electroencephalogram (EEG) recordings of "brain waves" (oscillations) provide an endophenotype for study of inherited traits. EEG recordings show four patterns of oscillations: alpha, beta, gamma, and theta. These are stable and are largely determined genetically. O'Connor and other investigators at the institute have participated in multisite EEG studies of alcohol-dependent individuals. In one study, DNA was assessed as well as EEG recordings. The GABRB1 gene on chromosome 4 was shown to be associated with the power of a beta oscillation. GABR genes are associated with GABAA receptors and beta oscillations in EEG. Fast synaptic activation is mediated by these receptors, which play an important role in response to alcohol.[13] The GABRA2 gene on chromosome 4 is associated with the GABAA receptor a2 subunit that regulates neural signaling (electrical activity of neurons) and is associated with increased risk for alcohol dependence, drug dependence, and conduct disorders. Another of the GABR genes, GABRG3 on chromosome 15, is associated with GABAA receptor g3 subunit, regulates neural signaling, and leads to increased risk for developing alcohol dependence.[14]

In New York Henri Begleiter, PhD, had demonstrated that a particular wave (P300), occurring 300 milliseconds after a stimulus (e.g., a sound), is lower in EEGs of individuals with alcoholism whether or not they are abstinent than in those without alcohol dependence. This finding has been used in multiple studies of the biology of response to alcohol. O'Connor participated in research comparing adolescent children of alcoholics (at high risk for alcoholism) with age-matched normal controls that had no close relatives with alcoholism (low risk). EEGs were recorded in both groups during a task using three visual stimuli. Subjects were required to press a button during one type of stimulus. The high-risk group of adolescent children of alcoholics showed lower P300 responses to the visual stimuli. P300 is determined by theta and delta oscillations. There was decreased theta and delta power in the parietal area of the brain overlying the limbic system (hypothalamus, amygdala, hippocampus, and other structures involved in mood and anxiety) after visual stimuli in the high-risk group, which might well be a marker for alcoholism. It has a basis in activity of the neurotransmitter acetylcholine, related to the gene CHRM2 on chromosome 7, which encodes acetylcholine receptor M2, regulates neural signaling, and is associated with increased risk of developing alcohol dependence, major depression, or both.[15] These findings hold out the possibility of predicting the development of alcoholism before an individual has begun to use alcohol. Currently, the best predictor that someone will develop alcoholism if they start to drink is a positive family history of alcoholism—and this is far from one hundred percent accurate.

The EEG studies discussed above are part of the Collaborative Study on the Genetics of Alcoholism (COGA) that John Nurnberger, Jr. played a major role in designing. Collaborative sites for the long-term study are at Indiana University School of Medicine, SUNY Downstate Medical Center at Brooklyn, University of Connecticut Health Center, Washington University School of Medicine in St. Louis, University of California at San Diego, and University of Iowa. Researchers at each site recruited alcohol-dependent individuals from inpatient and outpatient treatment facilities. They recruited controls (non-alcoholic individuals) from HMOs, drivers' license records, and dental clinics in order to obtain a representative sample of the population at each site. After initial assessment, they excluded subjects with severe medical illness, psychosis, head injury, medication affecting brain function, positive HIV test, or recent use of psychoactive substances. Study staff interviewed alcohol-dependent subjects, control subjects, and relatives of both with the Semi-Structured Assessment of Genetics of Alcoholism (SSAGA), a questionnaire that evaluates alcohol and other substance use, psychiatric and medical diagnoses, and social and family histories. Blood samples were drawn for DNA analyses.

Alcohol in the body is broken down to acetaldehyde, which is rapidly metabolized. Acetaldehyde is a toxic substance that produces a flush reaction when present in greater than usual amounts: flushed face, sweating, vomiting, and headache. If the enzymes in the chain of reactions metabolizing alcohol are abnormal in such a way as to allow the build-up of acetaldehyde, they serve as a protective mechanism against alcoholism. Individuals with the genes that are associated with such abnormal enzymes soon learn that use of alcohol leads to an unpleasant reaction and do not drink. These gene variants occur with different frequency in different populations (e.g., more frequent in individuals of Asian descent.)

Details of the Variants:

When the ALDHI gene on chromosome 4 is present, acetaldehyde is not broken down, and the toxic reaction occurs.

When certain variants of the ADH4 gene on chromosome 4 are present, alcohol is rapidly destroyed, and there is an increased risk of developing alcohol dependence.[16]

When the HTAS2R16 gene on chromosome 7 is present, there is increased risk for alcohol dependence.

When the DRD2 on chromosome 11 is present, it affects a dopamine receptor that regulates reward (pleasure). It may be associated with risk for alcohol dependence and habitual smoking.

The DPRKI gene on chromosome 8 and the PDYN gene on chromosome 20 involve the body's pain control (opioid) system and regulate aversion and reward.[17] They increase the risk for alcohol dependence and may be involved in heroin dependence and cocaine dependence.

Some of the COGA studies have addressed genes related to tachykinins. These peptides (strings of amino acids, smaller than proteins) have many effects in brain and body. As far as is known, there are five tachykinins in humans: substance P, neurokinin A, neurokinin B, neuropeptide K, and neuropeptide Y. The gene TACR3 on chromosome 4 belongs to a family of genes that encodes proteins that function as receptors for tachykinins. Studies of COGA subjects revealed seven SNPs in the region of TACR3 that are associated with alcohol dependence, especially severe alcohol dependence or cocaine dependence plus alcohol dependence. Pharmacological studies in rats had shown that substances that act like neurokinin B at the NK3R receptor decrease intake of alcohol and block some of the behavioral effects, suggesting treatment possibilities borne out by data in humans in the COGA research.[18] Variations in two receptor genes for neuropeptide Y also showed association with alcoholism. SNPs in the NPY2R were significantly associated with alcohol dependence, alcohol withdrawal symptoms, cocaine dependence, and alcohol plus cocaine dependence. SNPs in NPY5R were associated with alcohol withdrawal characterized by seizures.[19] There are ongoing efforts to categorize subtypes of alcohol dependence. These kinds of data are valuable in such definitions and will lead to better methods of devising treatment for each individual.

Physicians treating patients with addictions have long observed that individuals who are addicted to one substance might well become addicted to other substances. Psychiatrists have noted that individuals with alcohol or other substance dependence might well have other psychiatric disorders ("dual diagnoses"). The COGA project has addressed these issues. One study looked at marijuana, cocaine, and alcohol dependence as well as habitual smoking in siblings of alcohol-dependent subjects as compared to siblings of controls. If an individual had alcohol dependence, about one-half of the brothers and one-fourth of the sisters had alcohol dependence. If the individual was dependent on marijuana, there was an elevated risk of marijuana dependence in siblings. The same was true of cocaine dependence or habitual smoking. Rates for siblings were elevated only if the subject was dependent on the same substance. In other words, these data suggest that the individual with addiction to several types of drugs has several types of genes related to addiction. Rates for siblings of controls were much lower than for substance-dependent subjects.[20] Combined with the findings of many genes related to alcohol dependence noted above, it seems obvious that inheritance of alcoholism and addiction to several drugs requires many genes and gene combinations. There is *not* one single gene for alcoholism or one single gene for addiction.

Other COGA research examined the clinical observation that alcohol dependence and depression syndrome (changes in eating, sleep patterns, and physical activity; self-depreciation; difficulty concentrating; hopelessness; suicidality) often appear in the same individuals and the same families. Genome-wide studies evaluated individuals and siblings with alcoholism and depression, alcoholism or depression, or depression only. The results suggested "that a gene or genes on chromosome 1 may predispose some individuals to alcoholism and others to depression (which may be alcohol induced)."[21] Official diagnoses currently differentiate between major depression (without alcoholism or drug addiction) and "substance-induced" depression. These findings suggest that the two are related. Other genes are no doubt involved. In other research that compared relatives of individuals with alcoholism with relatives of controls, there was an increase in families with alcoholism or antisocial personality disorder, drug dependence, anxiety disorders (panic disorder, obsessive-compulsive disorder, post-traumatic stress disorder), and mood disorders (depression, mania).[22]

Newer studies continue the research with both animal models and humans. Alexander B. Niculescu, III, MD, PhD, who was born in Romania and trained at University of California, San Diego, came to the Department of Psychiatry and the Institute of Psychiatric Research as director of the Laboratory of Neurophenomics. He developed Convergent Functional Genomics, a complicated mathematical model that allows combining many data sources, for example cross-matching of P rat brain gene expression data with GWAS studies of SNPs from humans with alcohol dependence; blood studies from rats and humans; and brain data from rats and postmortem human brain data from online databases.[23] More candidate genes for alcoholism are being identified by Convergent Functional Genomics. These exciting research techniques make it possible to use all of the animal and human data in the same assessment of important genetic factors in disease.

Individuals with alcohol or drug dependence are all too often seen in a negative light. Until recently they were seen as sinners or weak individuals lacking willpower. This is understandable in view of the difficulties—even tragedies—caused by their behavior while using large amounts of addicting substances. Traditionally, they are not welcome in hospital emergency rooms by even the kindliest of doctors and nurses. Studies of the genetics and biology of these disorders counter the notions of willpower and sin. Treatment of alcohol and other drug dependence would decrease alcoholism and addiction, preventing related marital and family problems; improving workplace performance; decreasing the need for law enforcement and incarceration for drunken driving, illicit drug use and sales, and related crime; and making neighborhoods and communities safer and more livable. A current social issue is that there are just not enough treatment facilities to help all who need it, including reaching out to those dependent individuals who don't think they need treatment. Educating medical, nursing, social work, and other students and encouraging them to enter their disciplines with knowledge about alcoholism and addiction gained in research is crucial. The more treatments there are and the more effective and efficient they are, the better trained health professionals are, the closer we are to achieving the goal of decreasing alcohol and drug dependence.

If nothing else is clear about this chapter, it should be obvious that the causes and cures of alcoholism and addiction are complex. As with any other disorder, researchers are putting pieces in a giant jigsaw puzzle. As more and more pieces are discovered, it sometimes happens that the fit of the many pieces is different than initially assumed. But the more discoveries that are made of the different genes, chains of brain chemical reactions, and environmental events that go together to produce the disease, the more points of entry become available for targeting a specific treatment. The development of an animal model through inbreeding by Li, Lumeng, and their group; the subsequent neurochemical studies in McBride's laboratory; the human genetic studies of Nurnberger and the COGA project; and the EEG and fMRI studies of humans by O'Connor and Kareken have mapped out much of the biology of alcoholism and addiction. EEG findings are close to making it possible to predict who will develop alcohol dependence. Davidson's work has shown that, as is the case in most other psychiatric disorders, a combination of medication and psychotherapy works better than either alone. The more we know about a given disease, the more opportunities we have to design treatment. Medication might well be designed to arrest these illnesses. Psychotherapy and self-help groups such as Alcoholics Anonymous will still be necessary in the long run to help individuals who are clean and sober to get their lives together again.

Notes

1. T-K. Li, L. Lumeng, W. J. McBride, and W. B. Waller, "Progress Toward a Voluntary Oral Consumption Model of Alcoholism," *Drug and Alcohol Dependence* 4 (1979): 45–60.
2. T-K. Li, L. Lumeng, W. J. McBride, and J. M. Murphy, "An Experimental Approach to Understanding the Genetic and Neurobiological Basis of Alcoholism," *Transactions of the American Clinical and Climatological Association* 104 (1993): 61–73.
3. R. L. Bell, Z. A. Rodd, J. A. Schultz, C. L. Peper, L. Lumeng, J. M. Murphy, and W. J. McBride, "Effects of Short Deprivation and Re-exposure Intervals on the Ethanol Drinking Behavior of Selectively Bred High Alcohol-Consuming Rats," *Alcohol* 42 (2008): 407–16.
4. W. J. McBride et al., "Differential Effects of Ethanol in the Nucleus Accumbens Shell of Alcohol-preferring (P), Alcohol-non-preferring (NP) and Wistar rats: A Proteomics Study," *Pharmacology Biochemistry and Behavior* 92 (2009): 304–13.
5. T-K. Li, L. Lumeng, W. J. McBride, and J. M. Murphy, "An Experimen-

tal Approach to Understanding the Genetic and Neurobiological Basis of Alcoholism," *Transactions of the American Clinical and Climatological Association* 104 (1993): 61–73.

6. E. A. Engleman, et al., "Ethanol is Self-Administered into the Nucleus Accumbens Shell, But Not the Core: Evidence of Genetic Sensitivity," *Alcoholism: Clinical and Experimental Research* 33 (2009): 2162–71.

7. Z. M. Ding, W. Liu, E. A. Engleman, Z. A. Rodd, and W. J. McBride, "Differential Effects of Dopamine D2 and GABAA Receptor Antagonists on Dopamine Neurons between the Anterior and Posterior Ventral Tegmental Area of Female Wistar Rats," *Pharmacology Biochemistry and Behavior* 92 (2009): 404–12.

8. W. J. McBride and T-K. Li, "Animal Models of Alcoholism: Neurobiology of High Alcohol-drinking Behavior in Rodents," *Critical Reviews in Neurobiology* 12 (1998): 339–69.

9. R. Longabaugh, P. W. Wirtz, S. B. Gulliver, and D. Davidson, "Extended Naltrexone and Broad Spectrum Treatment or Motivational Enhancement Therapy," *Psychopharmacology* 206 (2009): 367–76.

10. V. Bragulat, M. Dzemidzic, T. Talavage, D. Davidson, S. J. O'Connor, and D. A. Kareken, "Alcohol Sensitizes Cerebral Responses to the Odors of Alcoholic Drinks: An fMRI Study," *Alcoholism: Clinical and Experimental Research* 32 (2008): 1124–34.

11. W. M. Pratt and D. Davidson, "Role of the HPA Axis and the A118G Polymorphism of the M-Opioid Receptor in Stress-Induced Drinking Behavior," *Alcohol and Alcoholism* 44 (2009): 358–65.

12. K. K. Yoder, C. C. Constantinescu, D. A. Kareken, M. D. Normandin, T. E. Cheng, S. J. O'Connor, and E. D. Morris, "Heterogeneous Effects of Alcohol on Dopamine Release in the Striatum: A PET Study," *Alcoholism: Clinical and Experimental Research* 31 (2007): 965–73.

13. B. Porjesz, et al., "Linkage Disequilibrium between the Beta Frequency of the Human EEG and a GABAA Reception Gene Locus," *Proceedings of the National Academy of Sciences* 99 (2002): 3729–33.

14. J. I. Nurnberger Jr. and L. J. Beirut, "Seeking the Connections: Alcoholism and Our Genes," *Scientific American* 296 (2007): 46–53.

15. Nurnberger and Beirut, "Seeking the Connctions"; M. Rangaswamy, et al., "Delta and Theta Oscillations as Risk markers in Adolescent Offspring of Alcoholics," *International Journal of Psychophysiology* 63 (2007): 3–15.

16. Nurnberger and Beirut, "Seeking the Connections."

17. Ibid.

18. T. Foroud, L. F. Wetherill, J. Kramer, J. A. Tischfield, J. I. Nurnberger Jr., M. A. Schuckit, X. Xuei, and H. J. Edenberg, "The Tachykinin Receptor 3 is Associated with Alcohol and Cocaine Dependence," *Alcoholism: Clinical and Experimental Research* 32 (2008): 1023–30.

19. L. Wetherill, et al., "Neuropeptide Y Receptor Genes are Associated with

Alcohol Dependence, Alcohol Withdrawal Phenotypes and Cocaine Dependence," *Alcoholism: Clinical and Experimental Research* 32 (2008): 2031–40.
20. L. J. Beirut, et al., "Familial Transmission of Substance Dependence: Alcohol, Marijuana, Cocaine, and Habitual Smoking," *Archives of General Psychiatry* 55 (1998): 982–88.
21. J. I. Nurnberger, Jr., et al., "Evidence for a Locus on Chromosome 1 That Influences Vulnerability to Alcoholism and Affective Disorder," *American Journal of Psychiatry* 158 (2001): 718–24.
22. J. I. Nurnberger, Jr., et al., "A Family Study of Alcohol Dependence," *Archives of General Psychiatry* 61 (2004): 1246–56.
23. Z. A. Rodd, B. A. Bertsch, W. N. Strother, H. Le-Niculescu, Y. Balaraman, E. Hayden, R. E. Jerome, L. Lumeng, J. I. Nurnberger, Jr., H. J. Edenberg, W. J. McBride, and A. B. Niculescu, "Candidate Genes, Pathways and Mechanisms for Alcoholism: An Expanded Convergent Functional Genomics Approach," *Pharmacogenomics Journal* 7 (2007): 222–56.

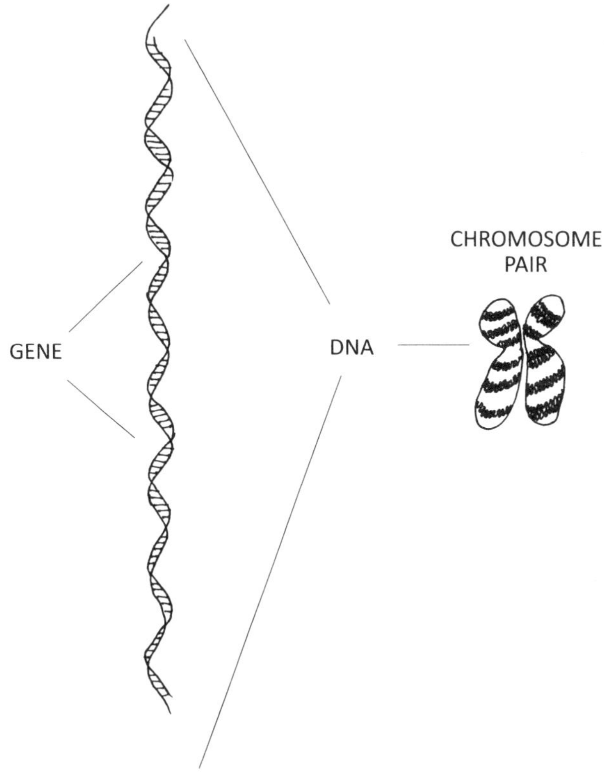

Each gene has a specific location on a specific chromosome and a mate ("allele") on the other chromosome of the pair. Gene are made of DNA (desoxyribonucleic acid). Chromosomes are double strands of DNA twisted into spirals (the "double helix"). Genes pass on their information to RNA molecules which ultimately bring about the formation of proteins which have multiple functions throughout the body. There are about 22,000 genes that code protein. [See pp. 102-3.]

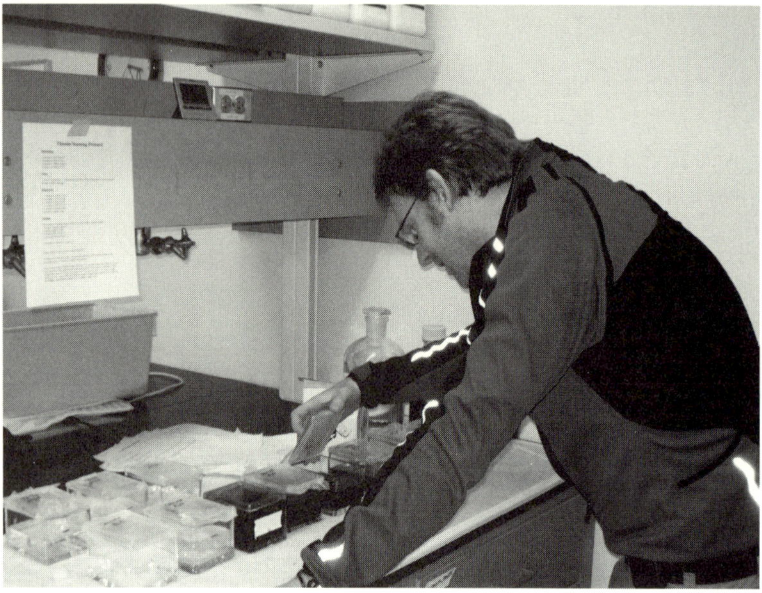

Researcher Dr. R. Andrew Chambers in his lab at the Institute of Psychiatric Research checking cell stains for brain tissue.

9
Nothing Is So Constant As Change
Larue Carter Hospital IV

For Larue Carter Hospital, which even today stands at its "new" location on Cold Spring Road, the twenty-first century has been characterized so far by significant contributions to the integration of the Recovery Model into inpatient psychiatry, the study of novel medication approaches to schizophrenia, and the introduction of partnership with an addiction treatment hospital for dual diagnosis services for all age groups at the hospital. It has also been marked by rapid turnover in leadership. Superintendents have been appointed and replaced at a much more rapid rate than at any time in this hospital's history.

When Diana Haugh left Larue Carter in 2003, she was only the fourth superintendent of the hospital. One of the authors, Alan Schmetzer, came to be her replacement, so it seems easier all around for him to simply report this portion of the history in his own words. His view is a window on the inner workings of administration, which is part of the mix for successful functioning of psychiatric hospitals—and general hospitals for that matter. It will also provide an interesting perspective on the issues, political, personal and financial, and the problems facing our mental health facilities as they attempt to address the disorders of citizens who need their services.

> At the time, although still full-time faculty at IU, I was the part-time medical director for the Indiana Division of Mental Health and Addiction. Suzanne Clifford was the division director for whom I was working. She, of course, was charged with conducting the search for the next Carter Hospital superinten-

dent who would replace Diana Haugh. This was a national search, much like the ones that culminated in the appointments of Drs. Nielsen and Moore. However, Clifford was finding it difficult to find the person she wanted to lead the hospital into the future. It wasn't that the applicants were not good enough, but she was attempting to attract "just the right person" while laboring under the usual state personnel issues of inadequate funding for a sufficiently attractive salary.

Although "waivers"—exceptions to the salary schedule—can be made, the negotiations to accomplish such changes take months, during which many excellent people who might otherwise have been recruited receive additional offers and often go other places. In any event, Clifford asked me if I would consider applying for the position. I didn't really think about it much at the time, but this may have been one way of solving her dilemma about the adequacy of an offer package for the position. My part-time work with the DMHA was a contract arrangement, and only about fifteen hours of my time weekly had to be paid by DMHA for my work. If Clifford could recruit me to the Carter position on a part-time basis, her budget would allow for someone with some built-in credibility (me, a tenured IU School of Medicine full professor) to be placed into the vacant position. That would, presumably, also make for "good press." My appointment also would be one Clifford was sure would be endorsed by organizations such as the Indiana Chapter of the National Alliance on Mental Illness (NAMI) and Mental Health America (MHAI) in Indiana, with whom she was trying to forge a strong working alliance. The executive staffs of both organizations knew me—I'd presented topics for each organization numerous times in my role as a faculty psychiatrist with the School of Medicine.

I never really expected to be appointed to the Carter position—there were, after all, several other really good people who had also applied if only a "deal" covering adequate salary could be worked out. I went through the usual round of interviews and appropriate "due diligence" with the other candidates. Clifford made it clear to me that my candidacy was, from her perspective, more than simple window dressing, and that in fact, she thought I could do the job if selected.

Nonetheless, it was still something of a surprise when she

called me into her office to announce that the search had concluded, and I would be offered the position. She wanted me to keep my position as residency training director for the IU Department of Psychiatry, just as Clare Assue had been a dozen years before. She made it clear that even though there were salary complications, I would be expected to do full-time work for a half-time job.

If I recall correctly, she did note as an afterthought that further contract money might be available later if my first year or two went well. I discussed the situation with the IU department chair, Chris McDougle. We decided that the benefits of having a superintendent at Carter who was closely tied with the School of Medicine once again—as had been the case with Don Moore and Clare Assue, for example—would probably outweigh the disadvantage of "deficit funding" for my faculty stipend. So off I went to fight the good fight, as it were, at an aging Carter Hospital that was embroiled in even more controversy than either the chair of our department or I had any notion, and we already knew there were plenty of problems.

One other fact I need to explain was that "contract people"—and that is what I would be on this job—are not supposed to supervise regular state employees. This is state law, and thus supposedly inviolate. The agreement with the American Federation of State, County and Municipal Employees (AFSCME) union to organize the workforce at the state hospitals had made much of this point, since many nurses and others working with the patients were not full state employees. At face value it would seem that I, as a contract person, could not supervise everybody in the system, as is required for the superintendent's position. But a way was found: the prevailing argument, as I understand it, was that Indiana University was also a state agency, after all, and that in essence an agreement could be reached for the president or board of trustees (or some such governing body) at IU to "lend" one of his employees to another state agency at the "pleasure of the governor."

Since the closing of Central State Hospital, the TV stations had been targeting Carter Hospital for on-the-scene reports about nearly anything that might go on there. This was a pitfall never dreamed of, at least in this degree of intensity, by Dr. Edenharter when his story of progress for mental patients through science began going out to the press. Central State Hospital was gone; Carter was the only institution for the mentally ill worthy of "investigative journalism," even though there might not be anything to investigate. I should have taken the press conference announcing my appointment as an omen of sorts about this new job: nobody from the media came to hear that better times were on the way for Larue Carter Hospital.

I'd been told that all the former superintendents of Carter had either died or been fired in office,[1] and I vowed that I would "change the luck" of the former Carter superintendents' "curse."

I knew all of the current psychiatric staff members from either my days in private practice or my presidency of the Indiana Psychiatric Society, and so they met me with a hard hat and some other hastily assembled joke gifts at my first medical staff meeting, knowing that Haugh had been having a very difficult time with both the external agencies and her own internal staff members prior to leaving.

Unannounced investigatory visits to the hospital by the Joint Commission (JCAHO) had become fairly routine at Carter. It may (or may not) have been that disgruntled Carter employees were calling the JCAHO with anonymous complaints. Even if those complaints were found to be substantively groundless, they caused endless headaches for the hospital's upper- and middle-level administrative staff as JCAHO staff members popped in and out amidst the day's needs for patient care and institutional management. Thus, there was a perceived need to get the employees on board with a united plan for the hospital's overall direction—and their part in it. At the outset of the administration of Governor Evan Bayh, an executive order had given state employees the right to organize. AFSCME had been chosen as the new bargaining agent for state employees such as those at Carter Hospital. Governors Frank O'Bannon and Joe Kernan had continued this arrangement. This meant that I had to work closely with union stewards on site to try to develop a better working environment for everyone.

I quickly initiated weekly meetings with union leaders at the hospital, made several trips to the union's offices in downtown Indianapolis, and established an "open-door" policy for any employee who wanted to come in for a chat. Soon the JCAHO stopped "dropping by" the hospital so frequently, whatever their previous reasons for coming.

However, just when my relationship with the union employees seemed to be solidifying, it was brought to my attention that the past decade had been one of administrative *laissez faire* in terms of oversight and structure within the hospital's business office. The prevailing philosophy of the times was that state employees would be better able to "just do the right thing" if a lot of the "bureaucracy" was entirely set aside in favor of "moving everyone around and stirring things up." Rules and regulations were seen as "impediments," and accountability, while still utilized as a watchword, became virtually impossible with the introduction of this new approach to running the "business of government." I knew even prior to the change of governing parties at the next election that a lot of "clean up" would be called for. The State Board of Accounts had to be involved, of course, and as a group these people are thorough to a fault. Audits and "plans of correction" were piled one upon the other in order to put the appropriate checks and balances back into place. And all of them had to be led by the superintendent.

I took over the reins at Carter in December of 2003.[2] In the middle of my tenure (although I wasn't aware at the time it was a midpoint) the governor's office changed hands from a Democrat to a Republican. This ended the agreement with the unions as spokespeople for state employees at Carter and was also the end of *laissez faire* business management. The new governor, Mitch Daniels, was a businessman, and he wanted all of Indiana back on a firm financial footing. I couldn't have agreed more, having been completely unable to tolerate the "administration by chaos" mentality described earlier, but of course the governor wouldn't have known this.

By this time, Carter was back to dealing with the JCAHO at arm's length, just like other hospitals, and the administrative structure was humming along in its former well-oiled "bureaucratic" way, which isn't always bad. I was dutifully trying to further the work of instilling a "Recovery" model in a state hospital,[3] a task Diana Haugh already had a head start in doing during her tenure at Carter. I met routinely with both the hospital's medical director, Jeffrey Kellams, and its clinical director, Timothy Lines, to make sure we were all on the same page in this endeavor. The DMHA was also working on an overall transition to the new Recovery Model by this time and had brought in Dennis Jones, former Indiana Mental Health Commissioner, as a consultant to move that larger process along.

Improvement in care for psychiatric patients is often surrounded, very predictably, by human issues and sometimes even made more difficult by them. The needs of patients in Larue Carter Hospital at the time were, of course, central to all parts of is mission, and all of us were trying to implement the Recovery Model to send our patients out to function at their best in the world if at all possible.

The Recovery Model is an excellent idea. It has seldom been really well defined, but most of us who work at it agree that it is based in concepts of respect and human dignity that recognize that those we serve and those who do the clinical serving need to work together on issues that are important to achieving the very highest levels of that person's potential for functioning.[3] Getting ideas directly from the person whose treatment is being rendered, family involvement, expecting good results, and celebrating victories along the way—all of these have been discussed as a part of the Recovery Model.[4] The model works best in outpatient settings, where there is more individual freedom. It is more difficult, but certainly not impossible, to instill this model into a system as old and hierarchical as a state hospital, where one needs a doctor's "order" written into the chart even to get up out of bed or go to the bathroom. But, things were moving along, or so I thought.

When I took over as superintendent, Suzanne Clifford had believed that I could do the job part-time if I had a chief operating officer (COO) working with me to help with day-to-day administration. After nearly eighteen months on the job, I finally got approval to hire into the COO position, and my top candidate was Lisa Kellum, a clinician-administrator who had previously worked with Midtown Mental Health Center.

Kellum came with great recommendations and had both a clinical (MSW) and business (MBA) knowledge base. She was able to hit the ground running, so to speak, and being from the community sector, was very much on-board with the recovery approach to, we hoped, improve Carter. It was in need of improving. For example, the main portions of the building to which Carter had moved from its original Indiana University Medical Center location on West Tenth Street were actually older than its original building. Some of the "new building" had been erected in the 1930s, and none of it had ever been intended primarily as a psychiatric hospital, although part of it had been built to provide psychiatric library, research, and outpatient facilities. Twice, including once during my term as superintendent, the State Budget Agency had been ready to release the funds for a truly "new" Carter Hospital to be built, and both times, economic downturns shut the door just prior to ground breaking.

The members of the General Assembly were aware that deferred maintenance from the days when the building housed a Veterans Affairs Hospital program (I was once told that $5,000,000 in plumbing repairs alone were needed[5] and the fact that so many outside doors (forty-one, to be precise[6]) were set into the old building that we could not even keep patients inside who were on "elopement" precautions, made the Carter building a newspaper story—probably a whole exposé series—waiting to happen. I kept pushing for a new facility, though, and one that would be part of IU School of Medicine, as Carter had been from the 1950s when it was first built.

Although Carter Hospital today is still one of the IU School of Medicine's "affiliated hospitals," it is not situated with the others or connected to campus by the elevated People Mover that runs between Methodist Hospital and the medical school campus. Former Carter psychiatrist Marvin Miller had fought the move to an off-campus site, terming it another example of out of sight, out of mind. While it is not that bad, Carter has gone from being the center of the Department of Psychiatry and its educational program and a partner with the IPR to more of an adjunct relationship, which is a huge loss to its patients and personnel, as well as to the School of Medicine. Carter's staff is still able to do a fantastic job of patient care. And having bigger grounds around the hospital has surely been welcome to the longer-term patients now housed there. Still, I was working for a new facility closely tied to Indiana University again.

I had been reassured repeatedly that, even though my contract with the state had expired by this time, December of 2005, it would be renewed. That had not happened, with various plausible excuses being offered, and the contract renewal had not concerned me.

In the midst of all these present and future plans, most moving forward successfully, on one December morning just prior to Christmas Cathy Boggs, the DMHA Director who had replaced Suzanne Clifford, stepped into my office to announce that "The administration has decided to go in a different direction" and that my contract would not be renewed. She asked the COO, Lisa Kellum, to step in from an outer office, telling me that Kellum would take over immediately as acting superintendent but that I would have time to move my personal belongings out.

And that was that, the end of the "Schmetzer Era" at Carter Hospital. It was the shortest superintendency on record, I think, until Kellum herself stepped down fairly soon thereafter to take a position at Wellpoint, the giant insurance and healthcare company headquartered in Indianapolis.

I still speculate from time to time on what happened. Systems were improved and functioning at the hospital, personnel issues had been well on the way to resolution, and management was relatively smooth. There were other replacements in hospital superintendencies at the time, and perhaps there was just some sort of housecleaning going on. At any rate, state hospital superintendents always serve at the pleasure of the governor, or whomever he designates to act in his stead, and accordingly, leave at his "displeasure." It was an honor for me to spend a little time, anyway, at the helm of what I still see as a premiere example of the best of Indiana's public psychiatric care, Larue D. Carter Memorial Hospital.

As I noted, Kellum was appointed acting superintendent immediately upon my termination from the position. She was kind enough to ask me shortly thereafter to write a letter of "goodbye" to the Carter Hospital staff for the hospital's newsletter. I have always been grateful to her for that opportunity. Working in a state hospital remains, even to this day, much like having a second family.

I went back to an addiction psychiatry clinical position. Shortly thereafter, following the resignations of several other psychiatrists, the adult psychiatry service at Carter was essentially filled with new psychiatrists. Interestingly, not too long thereafter, I was also recruited back to Carter Hospital, this time to fill in for the director of research. Anantha Shekhar, MD, PhD, had taken on the research program at Carter when Joyce Small entered retirement. Now, he was being recruited by the medical school to be the next Executive Associate Dean for Translational Research.

Upon Kellum's recruitment to Wellpoint, the state looked to Todd Graybill, MBA, MSW, as the next superintendent. Graybill had been brought to Indiana as a consultant to get Logansport State Hospital through a rough transition of leadership and some problems with Medicare accreditation. He had pulled that off well, and his "reward" was a call to move over to Carter Hospital and try to gain some stability there. His specialty has been his ability to move from hospital to hospital, taking over at a low point and moving the organization forward to a position of strength. He had been brought in originally to assist with the nuts and bolts of the Recovery Model effort, and now he was being called upon for his "move us forward" skills.

Graybill did as he was asked, came to stay at Carter for some four years, and did a masterful job of continuing the work started there by Juul Nielsen and nurtured so carefully by Don Moore, Clare Assue, Diana Haugh, and the rest of us. He understood Carter's somewhat unique position in the Indiana state hospital system, with its foundations in both the state-operated facility system and in academia. State policy makers don't know what to do with it, and politicians fret that it may cost them the next election. But without *some* program doing the work that Carter Hospital does, sooner or later we would all feel a great sense of loss—it is a research laboratory where new learning goes hand in hand with knowledge dissemination. This is translational research in the trenches, right down there in the muddy impasses of everyday misery and joy. And Todd Graybill understood that.

Graybill finally got to go to the State Office Building to start work on his own "translational" job, but he was able to leave the hospital in the capable hands of Lawrence Lisak, MBA, who had recently left a position as director of behavioral care at Methodist Hospital. Larry has been active in administering mental health programs in various not-for-profit settings and brings a true business perspective to the position for the first time, his background being an MBA. I expect a bright future for him and the facility as this book goes to press.

Carter Hospital's story has been one of trial and tribulation, at least "at the top." From the day Juul Nielsen first took up the cause of a "totally new mental health facility" in 1951 to Larry Lisak's tenure in 2010, as Iver Small, who was on the administrative staff for many years, puts it, "The place will just break your heart."[7] But it's in a good cause, and the improvement we get to see in the people who come to Carter for services makes even the heartbreak worth it to those of us who care about improving psychiatric care and humane treatment of the mentally ill.

Notes

1. Personal communication between Dr. I. Small and the author.
2. *Indianapolis Business Journal*, December 8, 2003.
3. L. Davidson, M. S. Lawless, and F. Leary, "Concepts of Recovery: Competing or Complementary?" *Current Opinion in Psychiatry* 18(6): 664–67,2005.
4. Substance Abuse and Mental Health Services Administration, "National Consensus Statement on Mental Health Recovery," http://store.samhsa.gov/shin/content//SMA05-4129/SMA05-4129.pdf.
5. Personal communication among various Engineering Department personnel at Carter Hospital and the author.
6. Ibid.
7. Personal communication.

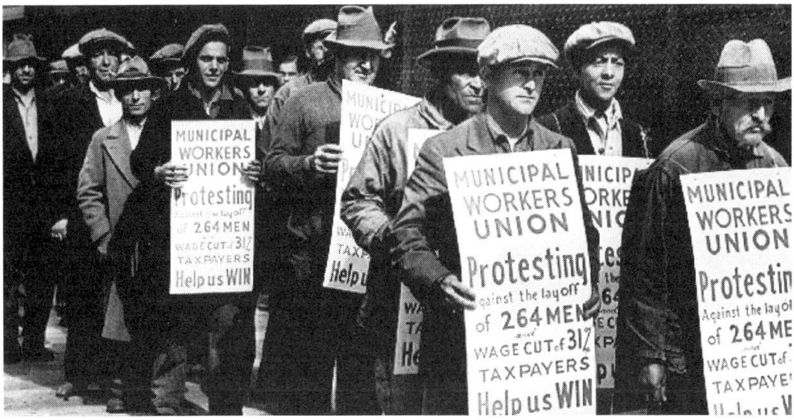
MUNICIPAL
WORKERS
UNION
Protesting
Against the layoff
of 264 MEN
and
WAGE CUT of 31%
TAXPAYERS
Help us WIN

AFSCME began in 1932, as the country suffered through a severe economic depression, when a small group of white-collar professional state employees met in Madison, Wisconsin, and formed what would later become Wisconsin State Employees Union/Council 24. Council 62 was formed in Indiana around the beginning of Governor Evan Bayh's first election, and became the bargaining agent for state hospital employees.

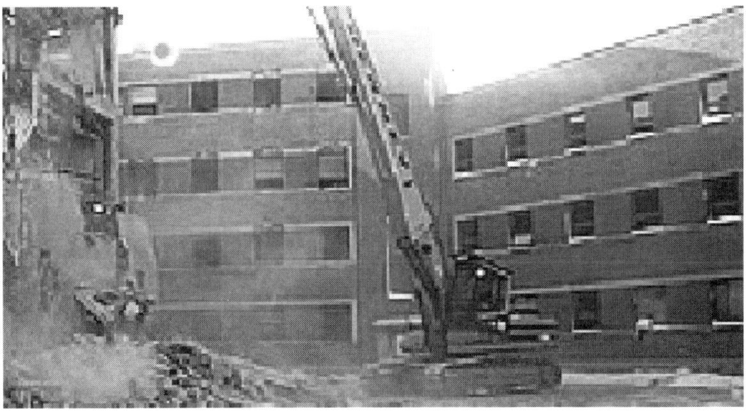

Time passes; changes come. To make way for the Wishard Hospital replacement facility, the original Carter Hospital building was demolished in 2010 by Denning Excavation Company.

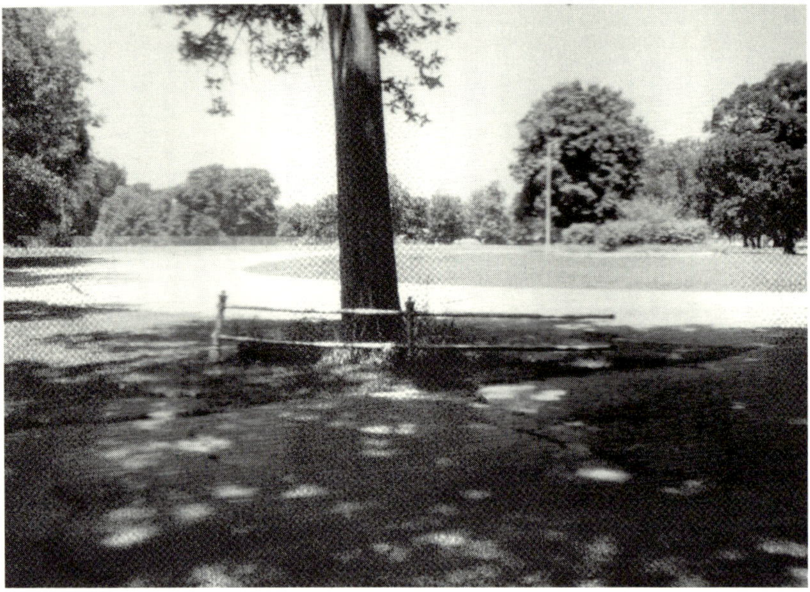

A fence in front of a tree is all that remains at the site of the historic Women's Building at Central State Hospital. Older buildings were progressively torn down with the closing of the facility, while some more recent ones are now utilized by the city of Indianapolis for offices.

10
Something Horrible Had Come Over Me
Disorders of Mood and Anxiety
Institute of Psychiatric Research IV

Mood Disorders

About a decade before Dr. Edenharter began his work at the Indiana Hospital for the Insane, a patient there described the sudden onset of a depressive episode:

> I sat sewing until quite late but. . .I never finished it! Something had come over me! I wakened the following morning bathed in a cold, clammy perspiration with an inexpressible horrible sensation as though falling into some dreadful place of darkness! I had not the strength to speak or move! And a cold shadowy something seemed settling down upon me—indescribable but altogether horrible!

She described mania as well:

> I had a so-called "period of excitement"—that of raving insanity. I was conscious of my inability to control myself! Knew I was screaming, laughing and praying without the power to stop.

The patient experienced "feelings of intense excitement of which [she] was compelled to give utterance of some sort. If there was a chair or anything within [her] reach that [she] could break. The paroxysm would soon pass over."[1]

This book has emphasized the many changes that have taken place in the past one hundred and twenty years in understanding and treating psychiatric disorders. The disorders themselves have not changed greatly. Diagnostic criteria used now in the *Diagnostic and Statistical Manual*, fourth edition, of the American Psychiatric Association are similar to those used by Edenharter, Bruetsch, and Bahr, diagnoses that had been based on criteria developed in Germany in the late nineteenth century. These diagnoses are based on a concept that goes back to the 1600s and a historically famous doctor in England named Thomas Sydenham. Syndromes (disorders) are characterized by *groups* of symptoms that occur together and have a common course and outcome. Although definitions of diagnoses change with new discoveries, having some standard definitions is important for both treatment and research. If one can't describe a particular diagnosis, how can it be studied and treated? We know a lot more about treatment now than Edenharter did. As a result, our patients more often improve and, when they do, improve more quickly. But, the goals of complete understanding and complete cure remain elusive. The Institute of Psychiatric Research and collaborating institutions are seeking to find the elusive answers to questions of understanding and cure.

Both mood disorders and anxiety disorders are common and make up the majority of conditions seen in psychiatric outpatient practice and private psychiatric hospitals. (Public hospitals treat more individuals with chronic illnesses such as schizophrenia and some dementias.) Sometimes they are "dual disorders," associated with substance dependence: alcoholism and addiction. Mood disorders include major depression and bipolar disorder, which is characterized by both depression and mania. Both major depression and bipolar disorder tend to be episodic. Episodes might be mild, moderate, or severe and last days, weeks, months, or even years. Bipolar I disorder is characterized by manic as well as depressive episodes. Bipolar II disorder is characterized by mild manic episodes (hypomania) and depressive episodes that might be severe. Some individuals have "mixed" episodes with symptoms of both mania and depression at the same time. Because there is so much variability in the clinical picture, it has been difficult to determine how many people in the population have a mood disorder: estimates range from about 7.5 percent to about 17 percent depending on the methodology of the research.[2]

The depressions of mood disorders are not just unhappiness or reactions to sad events. People with these depressions exhibit such symptoms as depressed mood most of the time; markedly diminished pleasure or interest in activities usually enjoyed; changes in appetite/weight, sleep patterns, and activity; fatigue; unrealistic guilt; difficulty concentrating; and thoughts, plans, and attempts at suicide. Unfortunately, the last are successful in about 15 percent of patients, most especially if untreated. A manic episode includes elevated mood and symptoms such as grandiosity, decreased need for sleep, pressure to keep talking, racing thoughts, hyperactivity, distractibility, and involvement in pleasurable activities that result in painful consequences (e.g., buying sprees, sexual indiscretions, and foolish business ventures that are uncharacteristic of the individual).[3]

Both kinds of episodes can be very disabling, but the disorders are treatable with medication and psychotherapy. As was shown in previous chapters, Morris Aprison at the Institute of Psychiatric Research studied the first antidepressant, iproniazide, a blocker of an enzyme that destroys serotonin. Joyce Small at Larue Carter Hospital and her group studied lithium and anticonvulsants that benefit mania and the next generation of antidepressants such as imipramine, one of the tricyclic drugs (named for their chemical structure). They continued their clinical research with medications that subsequently became available, such as still newer antidepressants that increase brain levels of the neurotransmitters serotonin and norepinephrine by preventing their reuptake from synapses back into neurons for storage as well as with newer antipsychotic medications that can minimize mood swings as well as benefit schizophrenia.

The researchers at Carter Hospital also evaluated different electroconvulsive treatments. Electroconvulsive therapy (ECT) remains of value in patients who have not responded to other treatments. These treatments are brief and are given to patients after a short-acting intravenous anesthetic and a muscle relaxant so that they are not awake and there is no muscular convulsion, only the increased electrical activity in the brain that is necessary for a therapeutic effect. There is transient memory loss after treatments, but it recovers as the patient returns to his normal life situation. Newer electrical and electromagnetic treatments are being studied and are available for those with intractable mood disorders.

To move beyond these now-traditional treatments, it is necessary to have deeper understanding of the complex genetic and neurochemical basis for these disorders. Researchers realize that mood disorders are more than disturbances in the function of the neurotransmitters serotonin and norepinephrine as was once thought. Here again genetic predisposition seems to be a culprit, and Indiana researchers have been pursuing this line of investigation and will do so in the future. [See pp. 102-3, 143.]

As coordinator and a principal investigator of the National Institute of Mental Health Bipolar Disorder Genetics Initiative, John Nurnberger, Jr., with Elizabeth Hayden, PhD, reviewed research from his and many other laboratories of DNA samples from large numbers of families, some members of which had bipolar disorder. Linkage studies indicated potentially important regions of closely linked genes (haplotypes) on chromosomes 2, 4, 6, 8, 11, 12, 13, 16, 18, 21, 22, and X. (Females have two X chromosomes in the twenty-third pair; males have an X and a Y.) Genes likely contributing to bipolar disorder are COMT and MAOA for enzymes that break down dopamine, norepinephrine, and serotonin; DRD related to dopamine; DAT involved with the reuptake of dopamine into neurons; HTR4 encoding a serotonin receptor that influences dopamine; and 5-HTT regulating the transcription DNA to RNA for serotonin. Serotonin and norepinephrine are associated with mood and anxiety, and dopamine regulates emotion and motivation. In addition, DISC1 is a neuronal structural protein and G72 interacts with an enzyme that affects amino acids, the components of proteins.[4]

The plot has thickened considerably since pigeons pecking

for food depended on their brain serotonin. There is now technology to study aspects of serotonin activity beyond what was available to Aprison and his colleagues. The gene 5-HTTLPR regulates processes involved with the transport of excess serotonin from the synapse back into the presynaptic neuron (reuptake). It has been found to have a polymorphism (more than one normal allele for a given gene locus) that increases risk for major depression. In one study of potential risk factors, thirty-nine children who had no psychiatric illness were shown a sad clip from a children's video and then given tests to ascertain the mood induced by the sad video. Children who were homozygous (the same allele of the gene on both chromosomes of the pair) for a particular allele of the gene showed greater negative processing of test questions than those with other alleles. The results suggested that a risk factor for later depression is that thought content is unduly gloomy when processing information related to sad topics. This was the first study to examine genetic vulnerability in the context of thoughts responding to particular stimuli.[5] Carrying on the tradition of the Institute of Psychiatric Research from the beginning, research about genetics is taking into account the environmental context for gene expression and the related behavior.

In the past couple of decades researchers have discovered that neurons are continually modified throughout adult life. Neurotrophic factors are proteins that maintain, and sometimes modify, neurons. Brain-derived neurotrophic factor (BDNF) attaches to receptors on cells and sends messages to direct cell metabolism. It has an important role in the survival, differentiation, and outgrowth of specific neurons. Increasing evidence has been accumulating that BDNF abnormalities are an important risk factor for bipolar disorder. Previous studies had focused on one SNP and generally had a small number of subjects. The Bipolar Disorder Genetics Initiative under Nurnberger's direction collected data from families with members who have bipolar disorder, recruited from ten centers across the country including Indiana University and a satellite center in Louisville, Kentucky. A whole genome screen was performed for 644 families that included 2,909 individuals. Two hundred fifty of these families were selected based on two criteria: all family members were European American (in order to have a relatively homogeneous sample), and DNA was available from both parents of one affected individual in each family. SNPs from the BDNF gene on chromosome 11 were studied. All the SNPs were in one area. There was evidence of association between bipolar disorder and the SNPs in BDNF, including ones near both ends of the gene. The authors concluded that the evidence "supports a role for BDNF as a pathophysiologic [altered function] factor in mood disorders."[6]

Nurnberger also participates in research led by psychiatrist Alexander B. Niculescu, III, mentioned in Chapter 8, using convergent functional genomics (CFG) to develop additional information about the genes associated with bipolar disorder. CFG involves combining data from animal models and human patients plus controls and assessing the accumulated information with Bayesian statistics. Bayesian theory allows combination of observed data and inferences about prior events that have not been observed and makes it possible to evaluate large amounts of disparate data from different sources. These investigators, using data from their own studies and those of other researchers, combined data from four GWAS studies, human postmortem brain gene expression, human blood cell DNA, and animal model brain and blood data.

The animal models of bipolar disorder developed at the institute included a rat model of extreme mood swings induced by methamphetamine and mouse models with "knockout" genes.[7] Knockout mice are produced by manipulation of an isolated early stage embryo, growth of its stem cells in culture, removal of the relevant gene from one of the cells, and implantation of that cell in another female for gestation. In other words, one gene is deleted. The model used included knockout of the clock gene Dbp. Clock genes are those that regulate day/night variation of body processes. Malfunction of these genes is involved in the swings in mood, sleep, and other body processes that are disturbed in bipolar disorder. These mice have decreased motor activity, less than normal weight, and a blunted response to stimuli. These depressive symptoms switch with sleep deprivation to a manic-like picture, a common observance in bipolar patients when deprived of sleep. This switch is prevented by valproic acid, an anticonvulsant medication used to treat mania.

Six candidate genes were found to be especially likely to be related to bipolar disorder. There were three clock genes: ARNTL, RORB, and DBP. The gene for myelin basic protein MBP seemed to have decreased expression in depression. Myelin is the outer coating of nerve fibers. BDNF, as in the research described above, was found to be relevant. Interestingly, the Alzheimer candidate gene APP for amyloid beta precursor protein also seems important in bipolar disorder. Altogether over fifty potentially important genes were identified. The authors proposed that bipolar disorder develops with a cumulative combination, not just of the same genes but rather the same gene families or biological pathways, with the addition of a stressful environment making the dysfunction worse or a favorable environment serving a protective function.[8]

Each of these genes serves a different function in maintaining or modifying brain chemistry. Finding genes associated with bipolar disorder indicates the many chemical reactions involved in the complex biological picture underlying propensity to mood disorders. Each discovery opens the possibility of a new treatment—perhaps even a new way to predict the illness and institute treatment early on. There is hope for those who have not benefitted greatly from existing treatments.

The importance of studying environmental context along with genetic abnormalities has been emphasized in much of the research described above. The role of environment is more complicated than it might appear. It seems logical that fearful situations would precipitate panic attacks in genetically susceptible individuals, and severe losses would precipitate major depressions in individuals genetically susceptible for mood disorders. In reality, severe panic attacks or major depressions can occur with no obvious environmental stressors and, conversely, individuals with these disorders can experience stress without developing symptoms. On the other hand, particular events might precipitate panic attacks or major depressive episodes. These often seem to be specific to individual patients, and possibly are more likely if they occur in young people. These are among the many kinds of questions being explored at the Institute of Psychiatric Research.

Anxiety Disorders

"I knew this one might kill me, but it wasn't as bad as a panic attack." The patient was in the Intensive Care Unit of a general hospital in the 1980s after her first myocardial infarction (heart attack), but it wasn't her first attack of severe chest pain and trouble breathing. She had had panic disorder for years. Panic disorder is not just anxiety about worrisome events. It involves recurrent frightening attacks, often without a precipitating event, and concern between attacks that they will recur. The attacks include a group of symptoms such as a pounding heart, sweating, a smothering feeling, rapid breathing, shaking, a choking sensation, chest pain, nausea, dizziness, feelings of unreality, chills or hot flushes, numbness, fear of losing control, and fear of dying.[9] Ordinarily individuals do *not* lose control, and they *don't* die in a panic attack. But, as the patient quoted indicated, they certainly feel like they are about to die.

The disorder, usually beginning in the teens or twenties and ordinarily lasting for a lifetime, has been observed for centuries. It is a common cause of distress and disability; epidemiologic studies indicate that as many as 4 percent of the population, more often women than men, suffer from the disorder. Multiple theories have been postulated to explain the cause.[10] Sometimes a busy emergency room physician, having established that a very anxious patient does not have a life-threatening illness, has hurriedly said, "Don't worry, it's your nerves." In a sense, that's true. The disorder is related to inherited brain chemistry. It runs in families. In the last half of the twentieth century, research has been carried out by numerous investigators, including at the Institute of Psychiatric Research.

A number of chemical substances can induce panic attacks in susceptible individuals: intravenous lactate (a chemical in the pathway of energy metabolism) and yohimbine, a drug that blocks an inhibitory norepinephrine receptor thus increasing norepinephrine release, raising blood pressure and heart rate and causing tremor. Norepinephrine produces many of the symptoms seen in panic attacks. Breathing 7 percent carbon dioxide can also precipitate attacks. Abnormalities in the regulation of the "calming" neurotransmitter GABA contribute to attacks. Benzodiazepines and barbiturates, medications that enhance GABA activity, relieve the symptoms of panic attacks.

Obviously the neurochemistry of the disorder is complicated. Recent research at the Institute of Psychiatric Research has pinpointed an important clue in the cause and treatment of panic disorder. During the past few decades, Dr. Anantha Shekhar and his group, including Andrew Goddard, MD; Philip Johnson, PhD; and Tammy Sajdyk, PhD, have begun to tease out the various elements of this puzzle. Like most studies at the institute, their work has used both studies of an animal model and research with patients. The animal model uses rats with microcannulas (tiny tubes) implanted into a specific area (dorsomedial) of the hypothalamus, the part of the brain above the pituitary gland that directs a number of hormones and other chemicals to keep physiological characteristics such as blood pressure and body temperature in balance. For five days, the rats are infused with allylglycine, an inhibitor of the synthesis of the neurotransmitter GABA (gamma-aminobutyric acid). Rats with decreased GABA respond to lactate, yohimbine, and inhaled CO2 with increased heart rate and blood pressure, appear more anxious in social situations with other rats and in maze tests, and exhibit "flight"-like locomotion.[11] Among the human studies, neuroimaging (MRI) research by Goddard showed that patients with panic disorder have deficits in brain GABA activity.[12]

Orexin (hypocretin), a substance that regulates wakefulness, vigilance, feeding, sexual behavior, and other basic functions, occurs exclusively in the same areas of the hypothalamus affected in the rat model of panic attacks. It was found that cells that produce orexin were activated (through expression of a specific gene, c-Fos) in panic model rats after exposure to lactate. When another gene (Hert) that helps to produce orexin was blocked by pretreatment with the relevant RNA, the panic response in rats given lactate was attenuated. Orexin receptor antagonists also blocked the panic response. In other words, the less orexin present, the less severe the panic attack. The authors concluded, ". . . our results suggest that the orexin system may be involved in the pathophysiology of panic anxiety and that orexin antagonists constitute a potential new treatment strategy for panic disorder."[13]

In addition to his research in psychiatry, Shekhar is director of the Indiana Clinical and Translational Sciences Institute (CTSI), a collaboration among Indiana University, Purdue University, the University of Notre Dame, and other public and private partners. The purpose of translational research is to translate research discoveries into clinical trials of new treatments, for example, using orexin research to develop new medicines for panic disorder.

Panic disorder was initially treated by the barbiturates such as phenobarbital and, after their discovery in the 1950s, with benzodiazepines such as Librium and Valium. Both groups of medications act at receptors for the neurotransmitter GABA. Both groups of drugs can be sedating and addicting. Some of the antidepressants benefit sufferers of panic disorder and are not addicting but sometimes have unpleasant side effects that are troubling to patients who worry excessively and have panic attacks. The research with orexin opens entirely new possibilities for treatment.

In addition to panic disorder, the group of anxiety disorders includes posttraumatic stress disorder, phobic disorders (unusual fears beyond what would be expected from the fear-provoking stimulus), and obsessive-compulsive disorder (distressing and repetitive thoughts and rituals). Some of the same areas of the brain are thought to be involved in phobias and posttraumatic stress disorder. Orexin might well turn out to be important in these disorders as well as in panic disorder. The introduction of serotonin reuptake inhibitors antidepressant a couple of decades ago proved beneficial to the treatment of obsessive-compulsive disorder as well as panic disorder and the other anxiety disorders. All these disorders are treatable with medication and behavioral therapy.

Another structure in the brain, in addition to the hypothalamus, that is associated with anxiety and mood is the amygdala. The responses of the basolateral nucleus of the amygdala are usually under inhibition by GABA. The stress-related neuropeptide CRF (a peptide is a string of amino acids smaller than a protein) is produced in the hypothalamus and stimulates release of another hormone, ACTH, from the pituitary and leading to release of cortisone, a "stress" hormone from the adrenal glands. CRF is also produced in the amygdala, resulting in anxiety-like behavior.[14] In contrast, repeated administration of Neuropeptide Y to the basolateral nucleus of the amygdala of rats was demonstrated by Shekhar's group to produce long-term stress resilience to tests used in their experiments to produce panic-like behaviors, suggesting a balance between CRF and Neuropeptide Y in the amygdala in determining responses to stress. Neuropeptide Y did not affect the hormones of the hypothalamic-pituitary-adrenal system.[15]

Finding ways to maintain such a balance in patients with mood and anxiety disorders would open entirely new possibilities for treatment. The work of discovery of genetic and neurochemical correlates of mood and anxiety disorders and translating those findings into benefits for individuals who suffer from these illnesses will continue as the Institute of Psychiatric Research laboratories are moved to the new neuroscience building.

General References

E. Passarge, *Color Atlas of Genetics*, 3rd ed. (New York: Thieme, 2007).

W. M. Bolstad, *Introduction to Bayesian Statistics*, 2nd ed. (Hoboken, NJ: Wiley, 2007).

Notes

1. Anna Agnew, *From Under the Cloud,* quoted in L. J. King, *From Under the Cloud at Seven Steeples, 1878–1885*, 2nd ed. (Indianapolis: Indiana Medical History Museum, 2008), chap. 3.
2. C. S. North and S. H. Yutzy, *Goodwin and Guze's Psychiatric Diagnosis* (New York: Oxford University Press, 2010), chap. 2.
3. *Diagnostic and Statistical Manual of Mental Disorders,* 4th ed., text revision (Washington, DC: American Psychiatric Association, 2000), 352, 356.
4. E. P. Hayden and J. I. Nurnberger, Jr., "Molecular Genetics of Bipolar Disorder," *Genes, Brain, and Behavior* 5 (2006): 85–96.
5. E. P. Hayden, et al., "Early-Emerging Cognitive Vulnerability to Depression and the Serotonin Transporter Promoter Region Polymorphism," *Journal of Affective Disorders* 107 (2008): 227–30.
6. K. Liu, et al., "Evidence of Association between Brain-derived Neurotrophic Factor (BDNF) Gene and Bipolar Disorder," *Psychiatric Genetics* 18 (2008): 267–74.
7. A. Niculescu, et al., "Identifying a Series of Candidate Genes for Mania and Psychosis: A Convergent Functional Genomics Approach," *Physiological Genomics* 4 (2000a): 83–91; H. Le-Niculescu, K. McFarland, C. A. Ogden, Y. Balaraman, S. Patel, J. Tan, Z. A. Rodd, M. Paulus, M. A. Geyer, H. J. Edenberg, S. J. Glatt, S. V. Faraone, J. I. Nurnberger, R. Kuczenski, M. T. Tsuang, and A. B. Niculescu, "Phenomic, Convergent Functional Genomic, and Biomarker Studies in a Stress-reactive Genetic Animal Model of Bipolar Disorder and Co-morbid Alcoholism," *American Journal of Medical Genetics Part B* 147B (2008): 135–66.
8. S. D. Patel, H. Le-Niculescu, D. L. Koller, S. D. Green, D. K. Lahiri, F. J. McMahon, J. I. Nurnberger, Jr., A. B. Niculescu III, "Coming to Grips with Complex Disorders: Genetic Risk Prediction in Bipolar Disorder Using Panels of Genes Identified through Convergent Functional Genomics," *American Journal of Medical Genetics Part B* 153B (2010): 850–77.
9. *Diagnostic and Statistical Manual,* 432–33.
10. North and Yutzy, *Goodwin and Guze's Psychiatric Diagnosis,* chap. 4.
11. A. Shekhar, S. R. Keim, J. R. Simon, and W. J. McBride, "Dorsomedial Hypothalamic GABA Dysfunction Produces Physiological Arousal Following Sodium Lactate Infusions," *Pharmacology Biochemistry and Behavior* 55 (1996): 2499–2556; P. L. Johnson, S. D. Fitz, J. H. Hollism, R. Moratalla, S. L. Lightman, A. Shekkar, C. A. Lowry, "Induction of c-Fos 'Panic/Defense'-related Brain Circuits Following Brief Hypercarbic Gas Exposure," *Journal of Psychopharmacology*, Epub, January 15, 2010.
12. A. W. Goddard, et al., "Reductions in Occipital Cortex GABA Levels in Panic Disorder Detected with 1h-magnetic Resonance Spectroscopy," *Archives of General Psychiatry* 58 (2001): 556–61.

13. P. L. Johnson, W. Truitt, S. D. Fitz, P. E. Minick, A.Dietrich, S. Sanghani, L. Traskman-Bendz, A. W. Goddard, L. Brundin, and A. Shehkhar, "A Key Role for Orexin in Panic Anxiety," *Nature Medicine* 16 (2010): 111–16.
14. A. Shekhar, T. J. Sajdyk, D. R. Gehlert, and D. G. Raommoe, "The Amygdala, Panic Disorder, and Cardiovascular Responses," *Annals of the New York Academy of Sciences* 985 (2003): 308–25; A. Shekhar, W. Truitt, D. Rainnie, and T. J. Sajdyk, "Role of Stress, Corticotrophin Releasing Factor (CRF) and Amygdalea Plasticity in Chronic Anxiety," *Stress* 8 (2005): 209–19.
15. T. J. Sajdyk, P. I. Johnson, R. J. Leitermann, S. D. Fitz, A. Dietrich, M. Morin, D. R. Gehlert, J. H. Urban, and A. Shekhar, "Neuropeptide Y in the Amygdala Induces Long-term Resilience to Stress-induced Reductions in Social Responses but Not Hypothalamic-adrenal-pituitary Axis Activity or Hypothermia," *Journal of Neuroscience* 28 (2008): 893–903.

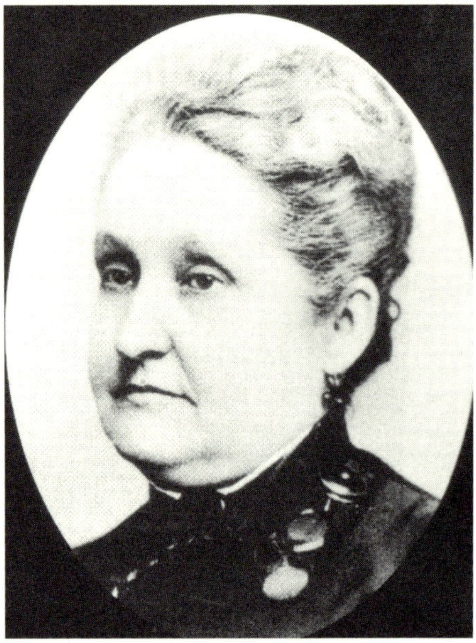

Anna Agnew suffered from what is today recognized as bipolar disorder. She came to the Indiana Hospital for the Insane in the late 1870s and later wrote about her troubles there in an age before much was known about the humane care of the mentally ill through science. From the book From Under the Cloud at Seven Steeples 1878-1885 *by Lucy Jane King.*

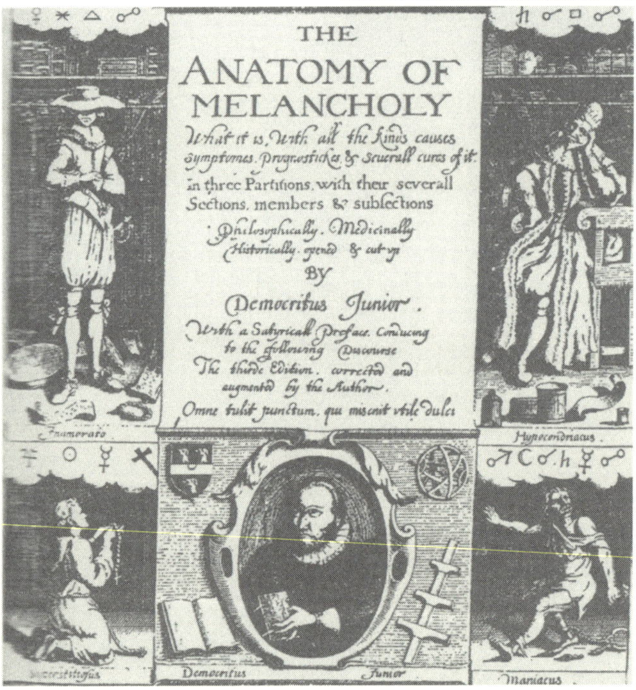

Mood disorders have been described throughout history. This is a section of the frontispiece of a famous book about severe depressive disorder, The Anatomy of Melancholy *by "Democritus Junior" (Robert Burton) 1651 in a modern (1927) reproduction of the book put out by Farra and Rinehart, Inc.*

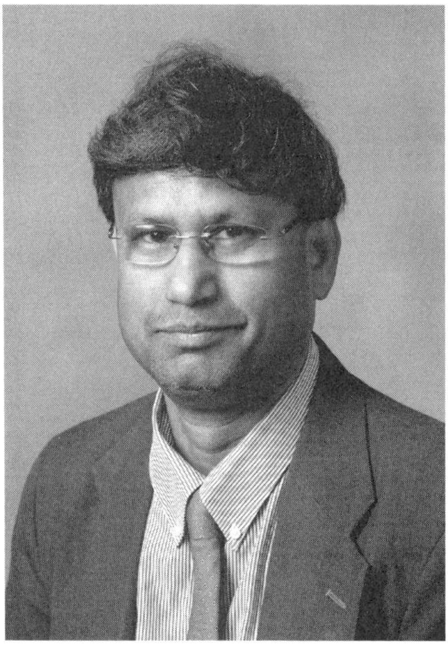

Dr. Debomoy Lahiri does research about the genetics and neurochemistry of bipolar disorder with Dr. Nurnberger, in addition to his studies of life-long contributors to Alzheimer's dementia. At least one gene seems to have some relationship to both disorders.

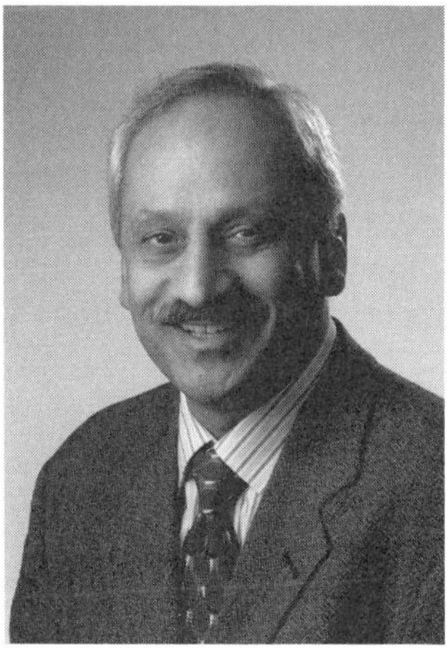

Dr. Anantha Shekhar studies both the basic science of panic, anxiety, and the clinical aspects of anxiety disorders. He is director of he Indiana Clinical and Translational Science Institute. Translational research looks for connections between laboratory findings and better understanding of clinical disorders and their treatment.

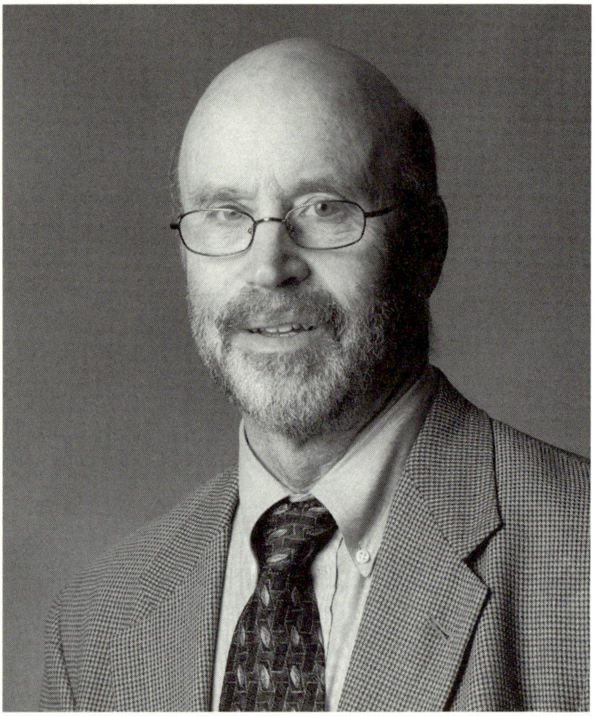

John Nurnberger Jr., Director of the Institute of Psychiatric Research. Photos of Lahirii, Shekhar and Nurnberger, Jr. are courtesy of Indiana University School of Medicine, Office of Medical Illustrators.

William McBride, using one of the best animal models of human disease, rats with alcohol dependence, mapped the brain chemistry associated with excessive alcohol use.

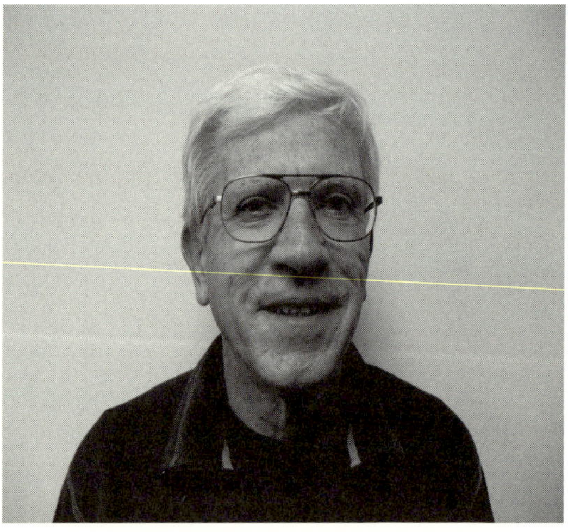

11
Educating Medical Students and Psychiatrists for the Twenty-first Century

A thread woven through the fabric of treatment and research described at length above is the third function of a medical school department—teaching. Educating physicians and student physicians was important to Edenharter and his many successors. All of the psychiatrists and scientists discussed in the book have spent time teaching first- and second-year medical students; small groups of third- and fourth-year students on hospital wards and in outpatient clinics; lecturing and doing small-group teaching for residents; doing individual supervision of residents about psychotherapy and prescription of medication for their own patients; or supervising research by medical students, residents, graduate students in the neurosciences, and post-doctoral fellows.

Psychiatry, more than any other medical specialty, requires the teamwork of many disciplines. Nurses, psychologists, social workers, and occupational and recreational therapists participate in treatment planning. Students and residents are involved as well. Patients express their own views and ask questions about their treatment. Both students and faculty members are constantly interacting with others within the psychiatric care community.

As the Institute of Psychiatric Research celebrated its tenth anniversary, the freshman medical student course in behavioral sciences, developed and taught by Nancy Roeske, MD, consisted of a one-hour lecture for the entire class, followed by ninety-minute small-group discussion sessions covering topics such as psychological effects of disease, patient characteristics through the life cycle, and working with dying patients. Drs. Toner Overley and James Simmons co-led the sophomore class covering defense mechanisms and their contributions to both healthy behavior and psychopathology. As in all other specialties, discussion of diagnosis and treatment are part of the training of medical students. The clinical clerkship in the third year consisted of a month of inpatient psychiatry and outpatient experience at one of the major hospital affiliates, as well as a half day each week during the outpatient pediatrics rotation interviewing a family at the Riley Child Guidance Clinic in teams of four students. Elective possibilities for seniors were expanded over the years to a comprehensive set of available offerings in settings scattered around the state.

In 1994 the behavioral sciences course was turned over to the Department of Internal Medicine, with psychiatry faculty still playing a major role in determining content. This change was part of a national movement highlighting behavioral studies as part of "primary care"—a controversial move. Many in psychiatry believed that with this new direction students would be shortchanged in their education about the psychological influences in health and disease. Indiana University, with freshman and sophomore medical classes located in nine centers, provided a natural laboratory for study of this question. About half of each class was assigned to the Indianapolis campus for the first two years of medical school, with the remaining half scattered over the other eight settings (Bloomington, Evansville, Fort Wayne, Gary, Lafayette, Muncie, South Bend, and Terre Haute). Indianapolis adopted this change first, followed by all of the other centers the next year.

One of the authors of this book, Alan Schmetzer, studied the United States Medical Licensing Examination (USMLE) behavioral sciences section scores for the first year class and found no difference in the scores between students participating in the primary care version or those who had received the more traditional psychiatry version.[1] These kinds of evaluative studies of student course plans are quite beneficial to faculty in planning best practices for teaching.

Psychiatry residency training was overseen for the first few years by the Psychiatry Residency Training Committee, chaired by John Kooiker, MD. Kooiker was in private practice half time and otherwise in the Adult Outpatient Psychiatry Clinic. He supervised residents in clinic in addition to seeing his own patients and taught the residency courses on psychodynamic psychotherapy using audiotapes, lectures, and discussion.

When Hugh Hendrie became chairman of the department, he felt that the training program's size and complexity warranted a training director. At the same time, the Accreditation Council for Graduate Medical Education (ACGME) was recommending that a specific person be designated for interaction with its Psychiatry Residency Review Committee. In 1976 Hendrie chose a young faculty member, Franklin Walker, MD, for this position. Walker's easygoing style of communication and attention to detail were just the right mix for moving the residency into its next phase. Residents now had regular feedback sessions with the training director. Individualized educational goals could be reviewed with each trainee. Walker served for three years before moving to a practice in Washington state.

Twelve new residents were selected each year in psychiatry. Funding provided through Larue Carter Hospital was supplemented by training grants from the federal government, where the National Institute of Mental Health (NIMH) was interested in having more psychiatrists trained for community mental health centers initiatives. Incoming residents could start after a year-long rotating internship (time spent in medicine, surgery, obstetrics, and pediatrics) the more traditional approach, or be accepted directly into psychiatry from medical school with the understanding that their first year would include six months of primary care, usually on inpatient internal medicine services.

In the 1970s and early 1980s, psychiatry residents' training at Indiana University consisted of two six-month blocks of inpatient rotations (including training in electroconvulsive therapy for six weeks), a six-month outpatient experience (including consultation psychiatry in other departments), six months of child and adolescent psychiatry (inpatient or outpatient), and three months each of community psychiatry and neurology. Lectures were held from four to six each Tuesday and Thursday afternoon on such topics as childhood development, personality theory, community psychiatry, history of the field, psychodynamic and other forms of psychotherapy, pharmacotherapy (use of medications), and diagnosis and treatment of psychiatric disorders.

When Walker left, Hendrie appointed Clare Assue as the next residency training director. She had supervised residents both on her inpatient service at Carter Hospital and in long-term psychotherapy and had taught several residency courses. Her charismatic teaching style was already well known throughout the department. For the next ten years, Assue not only was superintendent of Larue Carter Hospital, a story told in Chapter 7, but also provided leadership and direction for the residents. Clinical rotations were standardized, and lectures and seminars were consolidated into one afternoon session. There were growing clerical demands for residency training, handled by Assue's executive assistant, Brenda Carter.

It became clear to both Assue and Hendrie that the increasing requirements for providing and documenting residency training required preparation of the next director. Roger Jackson, MD, an excellent teacher from Midtown Mental Health Center, was recruited to be Assue's assistant training director. This appointment was prescient, as it was about this time that Assue was diagnosed with lung cancer and was soon unable to continue as training director.

During Jackson's time in this office, the requirements for both clinical rotations and lectures continued to change. Nationally, psychiatry residencies became four-year obligations without internship in order to give residents more time to mature as psychiatrists. Rotations in emergency psychiatry and in consultation-liaison psychiatry (work with other departments) were added. Even though the program had decreased in size from twelve new residents per year to ten because of decreases in federal training funds, Jackson found himself very busy, with a full service of patients at Carter Hospital and the complex training program to lead. The pressures of these duties probably played a role in his moving to Washington state, as well. The average tenure nationally for a psychiatry residency training director was about three years, and he served within that range.

Hendrie once again needed to recruit a new training director. He decided to look outside the department. John Vara, MD, was identified as someone who was a good teacher and interested in a move from the east coast to the Midwest, but he was training director at IU for only one year before being recruited to the Veterans Affairs hospital as medical director. Laura Reske, MD, had held the assistant training director position for a brief time before being named as Vara's replacement. Unfortunately she had not planned on moving into the training director role so quickly. She resigned from this position after only three months in order to enter private practice.

Hendrie had recently reorganized the psychiatry department into four separate areas, each directed by a vice chairman. After a stint as acting chairman during one of Hendrie's sabbatical leaves, followed by nearly three years as assistant chair to help with the administrative demands of the ever-growing department, Schmetzer was appointed vice-chair for education. Hendrie and he convinced Mary Landy, MD, to return from private practice to the full-time faculty to become residency training director.

Landy was a gifted clinician and a very capable teacher and administrator. She was able to quickly revive the residency after the previous rapid turnover in leadership. A very energetic and enthusiastic person, she involved nearly everyone else on the faculty to assist her by initiating projects to transform the didactic program and reorganize rotations to match the latest requirements laid out by the Residency Review Committee (RRC) for Psychiatry. She recruited a new residency coordinator and set about developing an organized approach to tracking resident rotations and accomplishments within a system for documenting their progress in real time. She also set up a smaller committee to develop remediation plans for residents who were showing signs of struggling in their learning. She was instrumental as well in developing a "Triple Board" (general psychiatry, child and adolescent psychiatry, pediatrics) option for residents requiring five years. This gifted leader also worked with the Department of Neurology to initiate a combined neurology and psychiatry six-year track. New post-residency fellowships were developed in geriatric psychiatry, under the direction of first Hendrie and then Valerie Smith-Gamble, MD; in addiction psychiatry, which Schmetzer led; and in research, directed by Anantha Shekhar. Training in research was deemed useful since Indiana still has to rely to a fairly large degree on "home-grown" psychiatrists for faculty positions, and Indiana University School of Medicine requirements for faculty were becoming ever more dependent on research prowess.

After three years of excellent work and a successful on-site inspection by the Accreditation Council for Graduate Medical Education, Residency Review Committee (ACGME RRC) in Psychiatry, Landy returned to private practice in 1998. Schmetzer was then persuaded to take over the residency directorship in order to provide continuity after the relatively short tenures of recent directors. A first-person account by Schmetzer himself will give insight into this period in education in Indiana's psychiatric institutions:

> Having learned from Dr. Landy's example that early and inclusive involvement of the faculty in the new director's plans was vital to success, I quickly formed teams to re-examine and revise the didactic curriculum and to develop new rotations to match the ever-changing RRC requirements for psychiatric training. As a lifelong educator, I looked to newly introduced ACGME objectives to inform the changes needed in both didactics and clinic experiences. Didactics (lectures and seminars) were organized by year; previously, lectures rotated in a cycle that had little to do with the timing of the residents' clinical experiences. We instituted didactics that matched concurrent clinical rotations. The first year of training covered the basics—emer-

gency psychiatry and the diagnosis and treatment of the major psychiatric disorders. The second year was about fundamental psychopharmacology and psychotherapy, with briefer psychotherapies covered as well as longer-term approaches.

The third year consisted of advanced techniques in psychotherapy and topics relating to collaboration with other members of the treatment team. Finally, the fourth-year didactics were focused on transitioning from residency to either fellowship or practice, with courses on such things as administration in psychiatry, business and budgeting, interaction with third-party payers, the ethics of involvement with the pharmacologic industry, and working with managed care and entitlements. There was also an academic track, developed with an emphasis on research and teaching, both necessary for residents who would be appointed to faculty at medical schools. Since Donald Moore's and Clare Assue's times, federal training funds had gradually stopped, and the residency education portion of the Carter Hospital budget had been frozen. The residency would be a victim of its own recruiting success if some way to fund the increasing financial burden of resident stipends, travel and book money, and insurance coverage could not be found. Additional training funds became available at this time through the VA system. Four new residency positions were approved, specifically targeted to a VA chief resident position, consultation psychiatry, addiction psychiatry, and battlefield "polytrauma" (the Army term for complicated injuries, both physical and psychological, sustained in war).

For the ensuing twelve years I remained as training director and steered the program through the transition from Hendrie's twenty-five-year tenure to a new chair, Christopher McDougle, MD. It was a priority for McDougle that a new assistant training director be identified. As part of his recruitment plan, he brought husband and wife, R. Andrew Chambers, MD, and Joanna Chambers, MD, to the IU faculty. They were both from the Yale faculty and had trained at the Neurosciences Fellowship Program there. Andrew

Chambers specializes in addictions and does research on dual diagnosis of alcoholism and addiction and other psychiatric disorders, as we've shown in Chaper 6.

Joanna Chambers had been in a leadership role in residency education at Yale, and following three years as director of psychotherapy education for the I.U. residency, she accepted the position of assistant training director. In this role, she immediately began to introduce ideas and promote changes that were necessary for the residency to continue its progress. The on-call system had become more and more burdensome for the psychiatry residents, and it became clear that a major overhaul was urgently needed. Chambers set up committees of both residents and faculty to try to generate proposals for change. During this process, the ACGME was continuing to amend its duty hours rules, so plans that seemed as if they might be feasible often had to be scrapped either shortly after, or sometimes even before, they were implemented. This is a process that could have become not only chaotic, but also very divisive to the department. Residents can feel "used by the system." Faculty, already pulled in various directions by clinical pressures, grant applications, and teaching responsibilities, are generally the only flexible workforce available who can be asked to cover if residents are required by ACGME rules to do less. Fortunately, Chambers had the fortitude and integrity to make the system work—eventually.

She moved into the training director position in 2010, and I stepped down to become her assistant training director upon retirement from a full-time faculty appointment. Chambers has continued to innovate. For example, there is a new "Power Hour" educational conference on Friday afternoons, which residents of all four years attend. Those sessions cover many psychiatric practice and administrative issues. The elective time in fourth year has been expanded from six months to twelve. New course offerings for the fourth year are designed so each resident can sign up for the topics that he or she feels will be the most useful in a future career.

Today education in psychotherapy has been turned around 180 degrees—residents now begin with cognitive behavior therapy (CBT) in their second year and learn how to listen to, and talk with, patients in very practical terms. Then, in the third year of training, they begin classes and supervision in psychodynamic therapy. This innovation came directly from resident comments and a study of how confident residents felt about doing psychotherapy.[2] The other didactics in year three are being changed to a "team teaching" format, so that several faculty members with various areas of expertise within a given topic will be present to comment and teach as the residents present cases. Residents have been encouraged to become much more involved in psychiatric research, both that being done by faculty and in their own original investigative work. In the 2011 Residency Match (the computerized program which places medical students into residency training slots around the country), Chambers was able to fill all seven available first-year positions.

The teaching portion of "Edenharter's dream" has been carried on intertwined with patient care and research, and all have been changing with the advent of new methodology and technology. As they move into the Neurosciences Center, their collaboration in change will provide hope to all those who suffer from psychiatric disorders.

Notes

1. A. D. Schmetzer, "Behavioral Science—Best Taught in a Psychiatry Course or a Primary Care Course?," *ADMSEP Newsletter* (Spring 1997): 6–8.
2. J. Bealke and A. D. Schmetzer, "Resident Psychotherapy Competency in an Age of Biological Psychiatry," workshop, American Association of Psychiatric Residency Training Directors Thirty-first Annual Meeting, Long Beach, California, March 7, 2002.

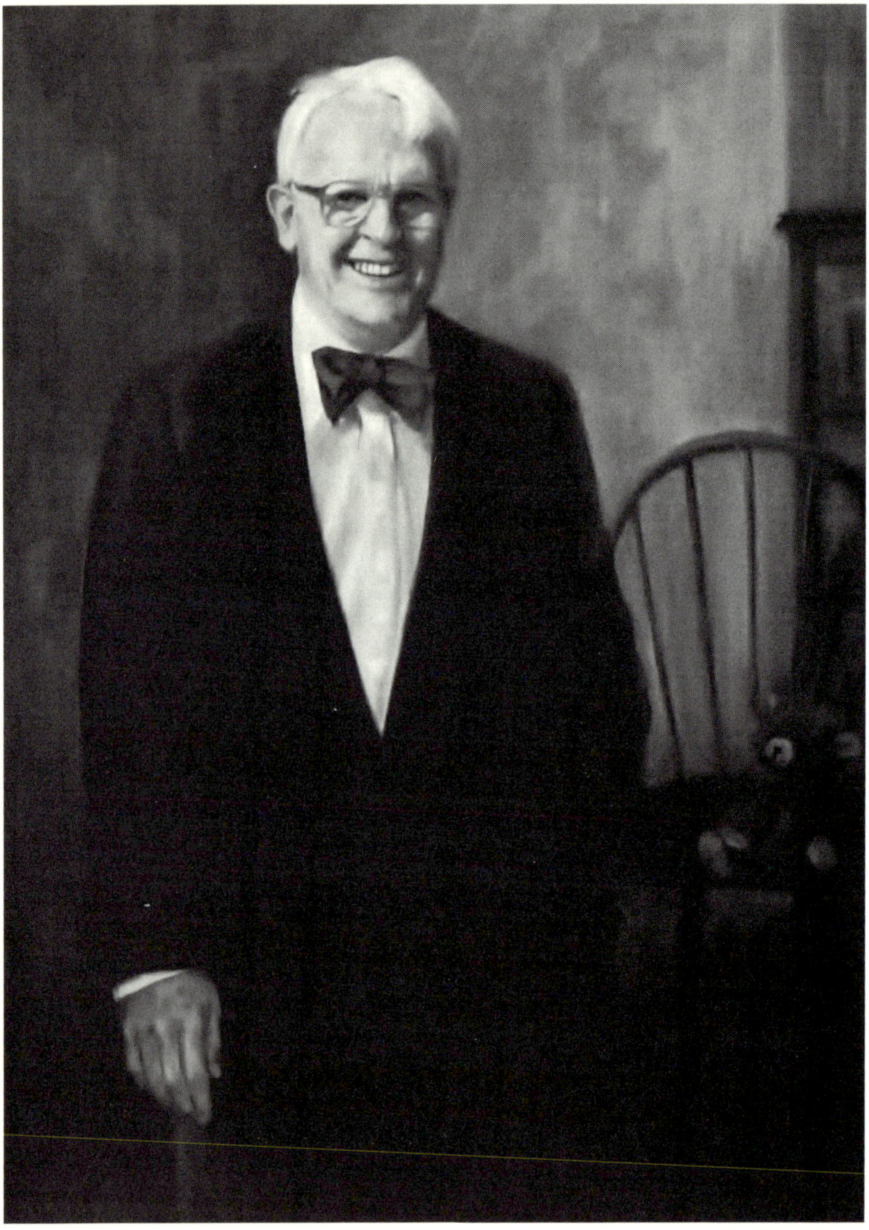

Dr. Richard Simmons put together a course for medical students.

12
The Dream Goes On
Neurosciences Center at IU

This book describes the work of hundreds of scientists and physicians who spent tens of thousands of hours working to bring new hope and possibly cure to our state's mentally ill through science. They, and their assistants, the workers who aided in the research and those who directly cared for patients suffering from mental illness, deserve the thanks and recognition we hope this book will generate. Physicians such as Margaret Morgan, Donald Moore, Juul Nielsen, and John Nurnberger, Sr., and after them Hugh Hendrie, Diana Haugh, John Nurnberger, Jr., William McBride, Joseph Hingtgen, Nancy Roeske, Franklin Walker, Anantha Shekhar, and Christopher McDougle have worked to fulfill the dream that reaches back to George Edenharter, at the Indiana Hospital for the Insane.

It was Edenharter's dream that his building and the concepts it represented would make a difference for the patients at the hospital and be a resource for those interested in learning more about psychiatric disorders. His dream, as we have seen, has passed on through work at facilities in Indianapolis and all across the state, serving over 100,000 patients annually today in Indiana, largely outpatient, with the best in psychiatric medicine.[1] The dream has transmigrated, strengthening into a network of research and care that has committed itself to the best in new facilities for our state in the second decade of the twenty-first century.

You may see a pattern in this story. First, Edenharter wished to establish integration of physical facilities for clinicians, researchers, and students not only close to the data, but also to each other, to interact and encourage knowledge and progress. A portion of this concept is now called "translational research," getting information from the "bench"—the term for the basic research lab—to the "bedside."[2]

We often hear about the explosion of knowledge in medicine today, and of how the sheer volume of information and the complexity of care have both become too much for any one physician, psychologist, nurse, social worker, or other professional, no matter how bright or how hard working, to assimilate and apply. So twenty-first century medical care is thought to be best provided by "teams" of healthcare workers who rely on electronics and other aids to assist in diagnosis and treatment and who rely on the kinds of scientific discoveries that require highly advanced technology that Edenharter could only vaguely envision.[3] All of this is true.

But we should look at the other side of the story. A truth that we do not hear as often is that all of medicine, but especially the field of mental health, has a long way to go in terms of *depth* of knowledge. Take any health problem, and any set of experts in that disease, and continue to ask for more explanatory detail, and you will eventually get to a point at which the members of your expert panel will look at each other, shake their collective heads, and say something along the lines of, "We don't understand that yet." The only difference in psychiatry is that this point occurs a bit more quickly in the questioning. Why is that? Well, the brain is probably the most complicated organ in the body. And, those working on the problems are using their own brains to study brain function.

Treatment, however, has of course improved spectacularly since the good doctor made his way from the wards of Central out to the quiet brick building in the corner of the grounds. Viewing a spectrum of those needing psychiatric help today, we can say their individual symptoms will respond to a given treatment at a rate of some percentage, very often somewhere in the range of 60 percent or so. But it is not good enough. Given the fact that we must rely on behavioral signs and symptoms, historical data from the patient and family, and a few non-diagnostic tests even to decide what we believe the patient's problem to be, mental health care does a reasonably good job today in assessing and treating the vast majority of people who come to us. It's just that those of us following Edenharter's dream won't be satisfied until we can do an excellent job for everyone.

Indiana University is making even further progress in this very direction. The new IU Health Neurosciences Center is the latest in Indiana's quest to solve these humanity-driven psychological riddles effectively and combines elements of the dream of humane and effective health care in our state in one facility with the best in physical plant and research availability, with even further consolidation and efficiency for best results in the plans for the future.

The events in this book have occurred in the Hoosier state. This state has not been known for jumping into controversy headfirst, but rather as a thoughtful, even conservative, part of the country. It is true that Hoosiers *are* generally thoughtful, and that is why they are also ready to roll up their sleeves to do things that support the arts and the sciences when they are convinced of their importance. Indiana has taken a leadership position in *how* psychiatric science and care should be positioned. The results so far are undeniable and have been shown in this book with breakthrough discoveries and in the recognition our researchers have earned nationally and internationally.

The next steps in psychiatric understanding will come through genetics and functional neuroimaging, or so we believe at present, and the Indiana University School of Medicine is well positioned to address these issues and advance the science of care. Scientist-clinicians in the new facility being opened as this book appears are deeply involved in this type of correlation. It would be the authors' hope that one day soon, when a person with a psychiatric disorder first steps into a treatment facility, he or she will have a thorough history and physical examination completed, a functional imaging study done, genetic and other simple blood testing completed and interpreted, and will then walk out of the facility with a full knowledge of the causes of the symptoms present and a treatment plan that is specific, complete, acceptable to that patient, easily explained to other family members, and nearly guaranteed to work. And if this comes about, it will be due in large measure to Edenharter's dream.

Notes

1. 2009 Community Mental Health Services Block Grant Reports (from Indiana)— "Table 3 Profiles of Persons served in the community mental health setting, State Psychiatric Hospitals and other Settings," accessed on September 25, 2011, http://www.in.gov/fssa/dmha/files/Table_3.pdf.
2. Khoury M.J. et al. The continuum of translation research in genomic medicine: how can we accelerate the appropriate intergration of human genomic discoveries into health care and disease prevention? Genet Med 2007 9 (10) 665-674.
3. Morrison G., Goldfarb S., Lanken P.N., Academic Medicine: Team Training of Medical students in the 21st Century. Would Flexner Approve? Academic Medicine, 2010: 85(2):254-259.

Acknowledgements

We are indebted to many colleagues who have provided material for this book. Among them are Drs. John Nurnberger, Jr.; Joseph Hingtgen; William McBride; and Iver Small. Judy Smith, former librarian at Larue Carter Hospital, and Frieda Cormack at the Institute of Psychiatric Research were most helpful with references, clippings, articles, and journals. *Psychiatry in Indiana, the First 175 Years* by Drs. Philip Coons and Elizabeth Bowman provided useful information about state hospitals. Clipping files at the Indianapolis Marion County Public Library central branch were invaluable as were the collections at the Indiana Medical History Museum graciously made available by Mary Ellen Nottage, executive director, and her staff. Pictures were obtained with the help of Michael Logar and Lawrence Lisak from Larue Carter Hospital, as well as Jan Royce. We are indebted to Nancy Niblack Baxter, Senior Editor, at Hawthorne Publishing for creatively making our medical jargon readable.